ORTHOPEDIC CLINICS OF NORTH AMERICA

www.orthopedic.theclinics.com

Education and Professional Development in Orthopedics

January 2021 • Volume 52 • Number 1

Editor-in-Chief

FREDERICK M. AZAR

Editorial Board

MICHAEL J. BEEBE
CLAYTON C. BETTIN
TYLER J. BROLIN
JAMES H. CALANDRUCCIO
BENJAMIN J. GREAR
BENJAMIN M. MAUCK
WILLIAM M. MIHALKO
BENJAMIN SHEFFER
DAVID D. SPENCE
PATRICK C. TOY
JOHN C. WEINLEIN

ELSEVIER

1600 John F. Kennedy Boulevard • Suite 1800 • Philadelphia, Pennsylvania, 19103-2899.

http://www.orthopedic.theclinics.com

ORTHOPEDIC CLINICS OF NORTH AMERICA Volume 52, Number 1
January 2021 ISSN 0030-5898, ISBN-13: 978-0-323-835-527

Editor: Lauren Boyle
Developmental Editor: Kristen Helm

Orthopedic Clinics of North America (ISSN 0030-5898) is published quarterly by Elsevier Inc., 360 Park Avenue South, New York, NY 10010-1710. Months of issue are January, April, July, and October. Business and Editorial Offices: 1600 John F. Kennedy Blvd., Suite 1800, Philadelphia, PA 19103-2899. Customer Service Office: 3251 Riverport Lane, Maryland Heights, MO 63043. Periodicals postage paid at New York, NY and additional mailing offices. Subscription prices are $347.00 per year for (US individuals), $1,003.00 per year for (US institutions), $411.00 per year (Canadian individuals), $1,028.00 per year (Canadian institutions), $476.00 per year (international individuals), $1,028.00 per year (international institutions), $100.00 per year (US students), $100.00 per year for (Canadian students), $220.00 per year for (international students). Foreign air speed delivery is included in all *Clinics* subscription prices. All prices are subject to change without notice. **POSTMASTER:** Send change of address to *Orthopedic Clinics of North America*, **Elsevier Health Sciences Division, Subscription Customer Service, 3251 Riverport Lane, Maryland Heights, MO 63043. Customer Service (orders, claims, online, change of address): Elsevier Health Sciences Division, Subscription Customer Service, 3251 Riverport Lane, Maryland Heights, MO 63043. Tel: 1-800-654-2452 (U.S. and Canada); 314-447-8871 (outside U.S. and Canada). Fax: 314-447-8029. E-mail:** journalscustomerservice-usa@elsevier.com **(for print support);** journalsonlinesupport-usa@elsevier.com **(for online support).**

Reprints. For copies of 100 or more, of articles in this publication, please contact the Commercial Reprints Department, Elsevier Inc., 360 Park Avenue South, New York, NY 10010-1710. Tel.: 212-633-3874; Fax: 212-633-3820; E-mail: reprints@elsevier.com.

Orthopedic Clinics of North America is covered in *MEDLINE/PubMed* (*Index Medicus*), *Cinahl, Excerpta Medica, and Cumulative Index to Nursing and Allied Health Literature.*

EDITORIAL BOARD

CONTRIBUTORS

AUTHORS

YVES ACKLIN, MD, DMedSc
Associate Professor, Department of
Orthopaedics and Traumatology, University
Hospital Basel, Basel, Switzerland

KOKEB ANDENMATTEN
Senior Project Manager Curriculum
Development, AO Foundation - AO Education
Institute, Dübendorf, Switzerland

CLAYTON C. BETTIN, MD, FAAOS
Assistant Professor, Orthopaedic Foot and
Ankle Surgery, Department of Orthopaedic
Surgery and Biomedical Engineering,
Fellowship Program Director, University of
Tennessee-Campbell Clinic, Memphis,
Tennessee, USA

KRISTEN A. BETTIN, MD, MEd, FAAP
Assistant Dean for Clinical Curriculum,
Pediatrics Clerkship Director, Assistant
Professor of Pediatrics and Medical Education,
University of Tennessee Health Science Center
College of Medicine, Academic Hospitalist,
Departments of Pediatrics and Medical
Education, Memphis, Tennessee, USA

ERIC A. BOE, DO, MS
Unite Orthopaedics Foundation, San Diego,
California, USA

MICHAEL CUNNINGHAM, PhD
Manager, Curriculum Development, AO
Foundation - AO Education Institute,
Dübendorf, Switzerland

DANIEL E. DAVIS, MD, MS
Assistant Professor of Orthopaedic Surgery,
Shoulder and Elbow Division, The Rothman
Orthopaedic Institute, Thomas Jefferson
University Hospital, Philadelphia,
Pennsylvania, USA

JENNINGS H. DOOLEY, BS
MD Candidate, Class of 2021, University of
Tennessee Health Science Center College of
Medicine, Memphis, Tennessee, USA

JOSHUA J. JACOBS, MD
Chairman, Department of Orthopedic
Surgery, Rush University Medical Center,
Chicago, Illinois, USA

TIMOTHY C. KEATING, MD
Resident Physician, Department of
Orthopedic Surgery, Rush University Medical
Center, Chicago, Illinois, USA

BASSAM A. MASRI, MD, FRCSC
Professor and Head, Department of
Orthopaedics at Vancouver Acute (Vancouver
General and University Hospitals),
Department of Orthopaedics, Complex Joint
Reconstruction Clinic, University of British
Columbia, Gordon & Leslie Diamond Health
Care Centre, Vancouver, British Columbia,
Canada

SAM OUSSEDIK
Clinical Director of Trauma and
Orthopedic Surgery, University College
Hospital London, Bloomsbury, London,
United Kingdom

CARSTEN PERKA, MD
Professor, Orthopaedic Department, Director
of the Center for Musculoskeletal Surgery,
Charité, University Medicine Berlin, Berlin,
Germany

FLORENCE PROVENCE
Project Assistant, AO Recon, Davos,
Switzerland

ARESH SEPEHRI, MD, MSc
Department of Orthopaedics, University of
British Columbia, Diamond Health Care
Centre, Vancouver, British Columbia,
Canada

JEFFREY M. SMITH, MD, FAAOS, FACS,
CPC
Orthopaedic Trauma & Fracture
Specialists Medical Corp., San Diego,
California, USA

CLAY A. SPITLER, MD
Associate Professor, Department of
Orthopaedic Surgery, The University of
Alabama at Birmingham, Birmingham,
Alabama, USA

KARL STOFFEL, MD, PhD
Professor and Team Leader of the Hip and
Pelvis Division, Department of Orthopaedics
and Traumatology, University Hospital Basel,
Basel, Switzerland

PHILIPP VON ROTH, MD
Sporthopaedicum, Straubing, Germany

ARISA WADA
Project Manager, Education, AO Recon,
Davos Platz, Switzerland

BAS WIJBURG, MSc
Senior Project Manager, AO Recon, Davos
Platz, Switzerland

RYAN WILL, MD, FAAOS
Olympia Orthopedic Associates, Olympia,
Washington, USA

PIPSA YLÄNKÖ
Manager, AO Recon, Davos Platz, Switzerland

CONTENTS

> Skills training is important in an arthroplasty curriculum and can focus either on
> "part tasks" or on full procedures. The most commonly used simulations in or-
> thopedics including arthroplasty are anatomic specimens, dry bone models,
> and virtual or other technology-enhanced systems. A course curriculum plan-
> ning committee must identify the gaps to address, define what learners need
> to be able to do, and select the most appropriate simulation modality and
> assessment for delivery. Each simulation must have a clear structure with
> learning objectives, steps, and take-home messages. Feedback from learners
> and faculty must be integrated to improve processes and models for future
> learning.

> Augmented reality (AR) technology enhances a user's perception through the
> superimposition of digital information on physical images while still allowing
> for interaction with the physical world. The tracking, data processing, and
> display technology of traditional computer-assisted surgery (CAS) navigation
> have the potential to be consolidated to an AR headset equipped with high-
> fidelity cameras, microcomputers, and optical see-through lenses that create
> digital holographic images. This article evaluates AR applications specific to to-
> tal knee arthroplasty, total hip arthroplasty, and the opportunities for AR to
> enhance arthroplasty education and professional development.

> The number of patients undergoing joint replacement and preservation pro-
> cedures continues to increase worldwide. Globally, there is no standardized
> educational pathway, training program, or recognized certification program
> for surgeons in these procedures. Development and implementation of new
> competency-based curricula to deliver specific educational events and re-
> sources may help trainees and practicing surgeons be able to perform these
> procedures more effectively and therefore improve patient outcomes in their
> respective countries. Ideally, a curriculum would be globally standardized
> and professionally designed to interactively meet the needs of surgeons. A
> competency-based approach with built-in assessment and evaluation pro-
> cesses is today's educational standard.

The growing epidemic of physician burnout suggests that a change is needed. Physician wellness is an ever-growing consideration, especially in orthopedic surgery, where the challenges to wellness are significant. This review provides many common sense wellness principles and solutions in four main components of wellness (physical, mental, emotional, and spiritual) interwoven with current research on the topic. Although directed to orthopedic surgeons, this guide can be applied to all physicians, because they are based on common human principles of wellness. Wellness is not created overnight, so wellness practices that increase the likelihood of experiencing wellness are encouraged.

As effective surgeon educators, we must seek continual improvement, to be "better today than I was yesterday." This pursuit of personal and professional development requires self-awareness of a guiding purpose, and grit, the passion and perseverance to achieve long-term goals. Surgical training draws on an apprenticeship model, where progressive transfer of knowledge, responsibility, and autonomy occurs over time as trainees work with experienced surgeons. Educators should model personal responsibility and technical excellence and require both of their trainees. While training programs shift towards competency-based learning, educators must remember that we shape learners with the "hidden curriculum" and not just the facts we teach them.

Professional identity formation (PIF) of medical students encompasses how students learn to think, do, and act as physicians. A key component of PIF is socialization, which includes mentoring. Mentoring influences students' career specialty choice, while providing a safe and nurturing environment to form their own professional identities. Mentoring of medical students by orthopedic surgeons may increase interest in the specialty. Suggestions for utilizing mentoring for the PIF of medical students and to increase diversity in orthopedics are discussed.

This article explores the current state of the residency match in 2020 with a focus on orthopedic surgery, analyzing the utility of current applicant screening methods in producing future generations of competent surgeons. Discussed are anticipated changes to the residency application process considering the COVID-19 pandemic and Step 1 becoming pass/fail in January 2022. Also explored are potential changes to improve the process for applicants and residency programs, such as identifying and using predictive factors of resident success in the applicant screening process, finding better ways to match applicants with programs, and increasing female and underrepresented minorities within orthopedics.

Over the past century, governmental involvement in the delivery of health care has grown steadily through health policy initiatives and increased regulations. Traditionally, the involvement in this process for the orthopedic surgeon was minimal because they were focused primarily on direct patient care. These two pathways have met a crossroads, however, where it has now become necessary for the orthopedic surgeon to advocate on behalf of themselves and their patients to guide and influence the legislative and regulatory processes. This article reviews the background of orthopedic advocacy and discusses ways in which the interested surgeon can become involved.

EDUCATION AND PROFESSIONAL DEVELOPMENT IN ORTHOPEDICS

SERIES OF RELATED INTEREST

Clinics in Sports Medicine
https://www.sportsmed.theclinics.com/
Foot and Ankle Clinics
https://www.foot.theclinics.com/
Hand Clinics
https://www.hand.theclinics.com/
Physical Medicine and Rehabilitation Clinics of North America
https://www.pmr.theclinics.com/

PREFACE

This issue of *Orthopedic Clinics of North America* provides excellent guidance for navigating problems facing orthopedic surgeons, from training methods for total joint arthroplasty to self-wellness and mentoring of younger surgeons.

Dr Sepehri and colleagues describe skills training in joint arthroplasty using simulations with such models as anatomical specimens and dry bone models. They emphasize that each simulation must have a clear structure with learning objectives, steps, and take-home messages. Feedback from learners and faculty must be integrated to improve processes and models for future learning. Drs Keating and Jacobs provide an overview of augmented reality in both clinical situations and surgical education. This relatively new technology uses computer-assisted surgery that is enabled by tracking functionality, system control software, and a human-machine interface. This system is becoming more and more frequently used, and this article is a valuable introduction.

Dr Andenmatten and colleagues discuss the need for the development and implementation of an international competency-based curriculum approach for training in joint arthroplasty and joint preservation to deliver specific educational events and resources that may help trainees and practicing surgeons to perform these procedures more effectively and therefore to improve patient outcomes in their respective countries.

In addition to providing the best possible care for patients, orthopedic surgeons need to be aware of their need for their own wellness. Surgeon burnout is increasing in these difficult times, and Dr Smith and colleagues provide many common sense wellness principles and solutions in 4 main components of wellness (physical, mental, emotional, and spiritual) interwoven with current research on the topic.

Other articles call attention to the obligation of orthopedic surgeons to continue their own education; mentor medical students, residents, fellows, and younger surgeons; and make sure the resident selection process identifies the best candidates with consideration of representation within the field of orthopedic surgery that better reflects that of the general population to provide the best possible care to patients. Dr Spitler observes that the pursuit of personal and professional development will help educators shape learners and that the "hidden curriculum" is equally important as a well-planned didactic curriculum. Dr Bettin discusses the importance of mentoring relationships in the formation of a professional identity in medical students, improving students' satisfaction, encouraging a career in orthopedic surgery, and perhaps improving matriculation of underrepresented minorities and women into the field of orthopedic surgery. Dr Dooley and colleagues give a snapshot of the current state of the residency match and discuss anticipated changes to the residency application process considering the COVID-19 pandemic and Step 1 becoming pass/fail as early as January 2022, as well as explore potential changes to improve the process for both applicants and residency programs.

Finally, Dr Davis reminds us of the importance of political advocacy in the current health care environment and the necessity for the orthopedic surgeon to advocate on behalf of themselves and their patients to guide and influence the legislative and regulatory processes. This article reviews the background of orthopedic advocacy and discusses ways in which interested surgeons can become involved.

Overall, this issue provides a wealth of information on how each orthopedic surgeon can bring about changes to our profession from personal self-care to national and international influences. We hope you will find suggestions applicable to your situation in the wisdom shared here.

Frederick M. Azar, MD
University of Tennessee-Campbell Clinic
Department of Orthopaedic Surgery &
Biomedical Engineering
1211 Union Avenue, Suite 510
Memphis, TN 38104, USA

E-mail address:
fazar@campbellclinic.com

https://doi.org/10.1016/j.ocl.2020.09.002
0030-5898/21/© 2020 Published by Elsevier Inc.

Surgical Skills Training Using Simulation for Basic and Complex Hip and Knee Arthroplasty

Aresh Sepehri, MD, MSc[a,b], Philipp von Roth, MD[c],
Karl Stoffel, MD, PhD[d], Yves Acklin, MD, DMedSc[d],
Sam Oussedik[e], Bas Wijburg, MSc[f], Arisa Wada[g],
Michael Cunningham, PhD[h],
Bassam A. Masri, MD, FRCSC[i,*]

KEYWORDS

- Orthopedic surgery education • Arthroplasty • Skills training • Simulation

KEY POINTS

- Skills training is important in an arthroplasty curriculum and can focus either on "part tasks" or on full procedures.
- The most commonly used simulations in orthopedics including arthroplasty are anatomic specimens, dry bone models, and virtual or other technology-enhanced systems.
- A course curriculum planning committee must identify the gaps to address, define what learners need to be able to do, and select the most appropriate simulation modality and assessment for delivery.
- Each simulation must have a clear structure with learning objectives, steps, and take-home messages.
- Feedback from learners and faculty must be integrated to improve processes and models for future learning.

INTRODUCTION

Although surgical training is constantly evolving, orthopedic surgical training programs are largely based on an apprenticeship model.[1–3] A surgical resident works under an experienced supervising surgeon, with increasing intraoperative and clinical responsibilities as the trainee advances through the program. The assumption is that at the completion of the training program, the trainee will be competent to perform orthopedic procedures independently.

However, recent years have seen a decrease in surgical residents' operative autonomy in essential surgical procedures across specialties.[4,5] This decrease has raised concerns regarding the

[a] Department of Orthopaedics, University of British Columbia, Vancouver, British Columbia, Canada; [b] Department of Orthopaedics, Diamond Health Care Centre, 11th Floor - 2775 Laurel Street, Vancouver, British Columbia V5Z 1M9, Canada; [c] Sporthopaedicum, Bahnhofplatz 27, Straubing, Germany; [d] Department of Orthopaedics and Traumatology, University Hospital Basel, Spitalstrasse 21, Basel 4031, Switzerland; [e] University College Hospital London, 235 Euston Road, Bloomsbury, London NW1 2BU, UK; [f] AO Recon, Clavadelerstrasse 8, Davos Platz 7270, Switzerland; [g] Education, AO Recon, Clavadelerstrasse 8, Davos Platz 7270, Switzerland; [h] Curriculum Development, AO Foundation - AO Education Institute, Stettbachstrasse 6, Dübendorf 8600, Switzerland; [i] Department of Orthopaedics, Complex Joint Reconstruction Clinic, University of British Columbia, Gordon & Leslie Diamond Health Care Centre, 3rd Floor, 2775 Laurel Street, Vancouver, British Columbia V5Z 1M9, Canada
* Corresponding author.
E-mail address: bas.masri@ubc.ca

Orthop Clin N Am 52 (2021) 1–13
https://doi.org/10.1016/j.ocl.2020.08.001

preparedness of new surgical graduates to independently perform these operations. Numerous changes have played a role in this decreased surgical exposure. The implementation of the European Working Time Directive (EWTD)[6] in Europe and the Accreditation Council for Graduate Medical Education weekly work limit[7] in the United States have reduced the potential training opportunities.

Despite orthopedic arthroplasty data generally suggesting that clinical outcomes are not associated with surgeon and trainee level of experience when appropriately supervised,[3,8–10] there are some data demonstrating an association between surgeon volume and training level in operative time[10] and implant malalignment rates[11] for joint replacement procedures, which has increased pressure on supervising surgeons to perform procedures rather than trainees, as their obligation to patients potentially conflict with their duties as educators.[12] The Bristol Enquiry Report states that "patients should not be exposed to surgeons at the start of their learning curves."[13] The learning curve can be described as an individual's performance level, as it relates to procedural exposure and case number. As experience increases, the trainee's performance reaches a level where they can safely and competently engage directly in intraoperative patient care.

This improvement has led to the development of novel methods of training residents and qualified orthopedic surgeons who are starting new procedures or further developing their skills. The use of focused skills learning and simulation earlier in the learning curve enables trainees to achieve a minimum threshold level of performance without exposing patients to unnecessary risk. Stirling and colleagues[14] summarized the main simulation modalities (anatomic specimens, synthetic bone models, arthroscopic simulators, and virtual reality [VR] and cognitive systems) and identified advantages and disadvantages for each. This review discusses various methods to surgical training using skills and simulation stations in orthopedic surgery. These techniques have various strengths and limitations, but all offer the benefit of reducing patient exposure to risk during training. In addition, the early experiences of AO Recon's development and implementation of skills stations into their international arthroplasty curriculum will be shared.

BACKGROUND: SURGICAL SKILLS AND SIMULATION STATIONS

Simulation training has been described as "a technique to replace or amplify real experiences with guided experiences."[15] The use of simulation in surgery is not new, with anatomic specimens being a long-standing "gold standard for technical skills training."[16] However, recent technological advances have allowed for the use of synthetic bone models and computerized simulation techniques to aid in training surgeons.

Anatomic Specimens

Anatomic specimens are regarded as having the highest "fidelity," or likeness, relative to the anatomy of live patients. This enables simulated learning of surgical approaches in addition to procedural technique. The focus in joint replacement training is frequently centered around osseous preparation and implant placement. However, surgical exposure and approach are essential skills, and specimens allow trainees to perform dissection of the soft tissues, which is not afforded by other simulation methods. Despite their high fidelity, in some jurisdictions, such as in Canada, the ethics of procurement of these specimens has been called into question.[17] As a result, educators in British Columbia, Canada are banned by law from purchasing such specimens, and only intact cadavers donated for this specific purpose are allowed, which severely restricts the availability of such specimens.

Despite the widespread use of anatomic specimens in surgical training, very few studies have objectively assessed the translation of skills learned to outcomes in clinical settings. Bergeson and colleagues[18] demonstrated that the technical error rate decreased significantly with increasing specimen exposure to thoracic pedicle screw placement. Specimen simulation training has been shown to lead to an improvement in the confidence of participants to perform a procedure independently when measured by the resident trainees and the evaluating surgeon.[5] However, the translation of joint arthroplasty skills from specimen simulation to a live patient setting has not been assessed.

There are limitations to cadaveric simulation, which reduce its usefulness as a universal training tool. Donor numbers and therefore specimen availability may be limited, and the associated cost with preparation, storage, and access is prohibitive in some countries. In addition, repeated freezing-thawing cycles have been shown to jeopardize the integrity of the soft tissues.[19] In joint replacement simulation, specimens are realistically limited to a single use following osseous preparation and implantation. This also means that simple tasks that benefit from frequent repetition for skill improvement, such as using a saw for example, cannot be practiced repeatedly on the same specimen.

Synthetic Bone Models

Synthetic bone models allow orthopedic surgeons to work on specific technical skills surrounding the bony preparation and implant application for joint replacement. Although the lack of any soft tissues limits the utility in training surgeons with regard to anatomy, surgical approach, and retractor positioning, the low cost and consistent bony morphology allow for high repetition technical skills training. Education using synthetic bone models has been praised for effectively developing targeted surgical skills[20] and to have similar effectiveness as skill training using anatomic specimens.[16] Furthermore, modifications in anatomy and bone properties can be used to mimic pathology such as malunion and osteoporotic bone. However, concerns regarding the similarities in tactile feedback between synthetic and real bone have been highlighted.[21]

Computerized Simulation

Computerized simulation ranges from computer programs that develop trainee cognition without development of physical skills to VR or augmented reality programs that combine visual with haptic simulation to develop motor skills. Advantages of computerized simulation include the ability to modify and adapt software to simulate numerous clinical scenarios. Cognitive simulation offers a lower-cost and easily accessible tool[22] for trainees to gain proficiency in the decision-making and surgical steps required in a procedure.[23] Orthopedic residents demonstrated a greater ability to detect errors in the surgical procedure for total knee arthroplasty following training using cognitive simulation compared with residents who were trained primarily using synthetic bone models.[24] However, the translation of cognitive to manual surgical skills has not been demonstrated.

Recent advances in computer technology have allowed for the development of VR tools in simulated orthopedic education. Most of the studies assessing the utility of VR in orthopedics are related to arthroscopic procedures.[25] Simulations in arthroscopy frequently use the combination of computerized visual and haptic feedback. This provides an environment to develop instrument handling and triangulation skills without risk of iatrogenic injury on a patient. Furthermore, computerized arthroscopic simulation also allows for objective assessment of technical skills and has been demonstrated

to distinguish between experience and novice surgeons.[26–28]

There is, however, a lack of literature assessing the effectiveness of developing technical skills in open procedures.[29] Immersive VR is a novel development involving the use of a head-mounted display, providing a 3-dimensional environment, in combination with hand controllers providing haptic feedback. This development increases the fidelity of computerized simulations and allows for increased engagement from the learner. Lohre and colleagues[30] performed a randomized control trial assessing technical skills of learners on a cadaveric model following an immersive VR learning module on glenoid exposure for shoulder arthroplasty. They found that the immersive VR group had a decreased time to glenoid exposure and improved instrument handling.

THE AO RECON EXPERIENCE IN HIP AND KNEE ARTHROPLASTY AND REVISION FOR PERIPROSTHETIC FRACTURES

AO Recon is a global education organization. In 2014, AO Recon developed an international competency-based curriculum in hip and knee arthroplasty, with the addition of periprosthetic fractures, including revision arthroplasty, in 2016. They designed courses through a reverse planning process and started delivering these events from 2015. Competencies and learning objectives were defined, and a combination of education methods were selected (lectures in the form of presentations, case-based lectures, and small group discussions). Expert faculty were invited and several 2-day courses were delivered in many countries in most regions of the world over the first 2 years. These courses covered primary total hip and knee arthroplasty as well as revision and complex primary arthroplasty in just 2 days for participants with varying levels of expertise. Analysis of participant and faculty evaluation data and feedback from these events suggested the content covered was too broad to optimally meet the differing needs of a heterogeneous audience.

AO Recon's hip and knee curriculum taskforce and Education Forum analyzed the data and approved the separation of content and designed distinct "Principles" and "Complex" courses. The goal of the Principles course was updated to "teach the fundamental principles and current concepts in the treatment of patients with a need for primary arthroplasty in the hip and knee" and the target audience was defined as "advanced surgical trainees and newly certified orthopedic surgeons". The goal of the Complex course was updated to "teach advanced principles and current concepts in the treatment of patients with a need for revision or complex primary arthroplasty in the hip and knee" and the target audience was defined as "certified, experienced orthopedic surgeons who wish to enhance their knowledge and skills." Analysis of the participant and faculty feedback from evaluations of the past courses also identified 2 recurring themes related to skills: "add practical exercises" and "add anatomic specimen laboratory time."

In January 2017, the hip and knee curriculum taskforce reviewed the list of procedures in the curriculum and updated the intended level of outcomes for each procedure for the target audiences in both the "Principles" and "Complex" courses. Each procedure was assigned to educational categories of "Knows," "Knows How," or "Shows How." Procedures categorized as "Shows How" were analyzed in more depth because these would be the focus of the skills training through simulation. For each one, a decision was made as to whether the entire procedure should be covered or whether it could be broken down into key parts. These could then be addressed in dedicated part-task stations by whichever type of simulation would be most appropriate (dry bone skills station, practical exercise, or anatomic specimen). The taskforce and the education forum approved the design and integration of skills laboratory stations for both hip and knee arthroplasty into the Principles Course. A taskforce of surgeons was appointed to work on the new project, and a support team and resources were allocated. In January 2018, the taskforce and the education forum approved the design and integration of hip and knee procedures in the Complex Course. In a similar process, the periprosthetic fractures curriculum taskforce identified procedures and tasks for their curriculum to be developed in 2017, and a group of content experts on joint preservation identified procedures and tasks to be developed in 2021.

Based on a hypothesis that the addition of skills training would enhance each of the courses, dedicated teams of surgeon faculty were invited to develop and implement new activities. Each group was supported by a team and applied processes based on established adult education principles in curriculum development, instructional design, and Design Thinking. In this article, the authors share our experiences and describe some of the challenges and solutions and contribute their results to this field of education.

Design

A team consisting of one or more experienced orthopedic surgeons, some target learners, a curriculum developer, bone model developer, implant provider, and efficiency designer was assembled and held a series of face-to-face half-day meetings for each step of the process. They first had to decide what to teach based on an analysis of each procedure along with feedback from senior faculty. The surgeons identified challenging parts of each procedure that have "teachable moments" for learners starting to perform these operations. They then defined learning objectives, all the steps that would be completed, and the take-home messages. Finally, they had to decide how to teach the skill and select from a range of options—skills station for "part tasks" or full procedures using dry bone practical exercises, anatomic specimen laboratory, or another type of simulation—and how to assess the performance.

Development

During the first meeting, an overall concept was outlined. The design team developed models and stations based on the first idea, and a series of prototypes was tested with the faculty and then with target learners. Adjustments were made after each iteration of testing to ensure efficient and safe simulations were finalized using dry bone models, real and 3-D printed instruments, and assessment tools. Once the pilot versions were validated, the final models and stations and all the support documentation were created.

Implementation

For each new activity, a timeslot was scheduled into the course program, and adjustments were made based on the required facilities, transfer time, etc. A video was recorded for each station and exercise to help prepare the faculty and to use as a demonstration of what participants needed to do. Time was also added into the faculty precourse meeting to ensure all surgeons were able to moderate and support the completion of the new activities. A booklet was prepared for participants, and a guide and videos were prepared for faculty. Before each course, the participants were asked to rate their own present and desired levels of ability for each of the competencies, including performing the procedures. During each event, content usefulness and faculty performance ratings were gathered, and feedback was documented from participants and faculty regarding what went well and what could be done differently next time. In 2019, a needs assessment was conducted to help identify the needs of learners and to help planning to meet those needs.

Output and Findings

Over 4 years, simulations for more than 30 full procedures or part tasks have been developed, and many have already been implemented and evaluated in courses (Fig. 1, Table 1). Four of the skills laboratory stations and one periprosthetic fractures station have assessment tools integrated (Table 2).

AO Recon Principles Course

For the AO Recon Principles course, 6 hands-on stations for hip and knee have been integrated as half-hour educational experiences with a rotation plan for groups of participants along with 2 stations on templating a total hip and a total knee arthroplasty procedure. These skills stations have been used by 446 participants at 10 courses worldwide during 2018 and 2019. Using a scale of 1 to 5 (1 = Not at all useful, 5 = Extremely useful), they had an overall average evaluation rating of

4.64 (range 4.71–4.57) compared with 4.56 for lectures (4.75–4.38) and 4.64 for discussion groups (4.83–4.44). Ratings for individual stations ranged from 4.71 to 4.57, and the average for all stations at an individual course ranged from 4.89 to 4.39. A comparison of evaluation ratings for 3 key questions from 26 events in different countries from 2017 to 2019 showed better ratings for the 10 courses that included the skills laboratory stations compared with 16 courses that had no such stations.

AO Recon Complex Course and AO Recon/ AO Trauma Periprosthetic Fracture Course

The dry bone and anatomic specimen procedures for complex hip and knee and periprosthetic fractures (both revision and internal fixation) have been delivered in a smaller number of events in a range of countries in Asia Pacific, Europe, Middle East, and Latin America (see Table 1). Early feedback and evaluation ratings have been positive, and the models and exercise timings have been adjusted to optimize the learning experience to focus on key principles. New procedures continue to be updated and added every year. The latest plans include the design of arthroscopy, osteotomy, and other

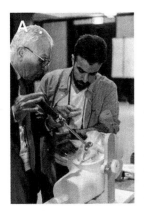
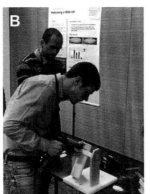
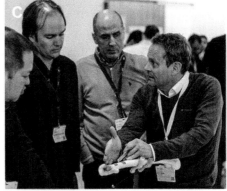
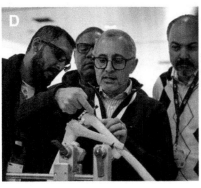
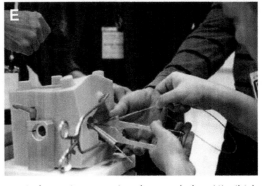

Fig. 1. Examples of AO Recon Skills stations and practical exercises: reaming the acetabulum (*A*), tibial cut (*B*), femoral stem revision (*C*), knee revision (*D*), and fixation techniques for periprosthetic fractures (*E*).

Table 1
Arthroplasty procedures to be delivered at a "shows-how" level from the curriculum

Procedure (by Course Type)	Dry Bone Practical Exercises			Anatomic Specimen Laboratory		
	Type	Time	Rating	Type	Time	Rating
Principles of total arthroplasty: hip						
Plan a THA (templating, etc)	Skills station	30	4.57	-	-	-
Ream the acetabulum, insert a cup	Skills station	30	4.71	-	-	-
Prepare the femur, insert stem	Skills station	30	4.69	-	-	-
Identify safe zones for screw insertion	Skills station	30	4.63	-	-	-
Screw insertion	In development	30	-	-	-	-
Primary THA	-	-	-	Procedure	TBD	-
Principles of total arthroplasty: knee						
Plan a TKA (templating, etc)	Skills station	30	4.66	-	-	-
Align for a tibial cut	Skills station	30	4.63	-	-	-
Perform a tibial cut	Skills station	30	4.63	-	-	-
Cementing	Skills station	30	4.57	-	-	-
Primary TKA	-	-	-	Procedure	TBD	-
Complex total arthroplasty: hip						
Posterior approach to the hip	-	-	-	Approach	30	4.50
Plate osteosynthesis of the posterior column	Procedure	15	4.38	Procedure	Option	-
Remove a well-integrated hemispherical cup	Procedure	15	4.63	-	-	-
Implant a hemispherical revision cup	Procedure	40	4.67	Procedure	80	4.59
Extended trochanteric osteotomy (ETO)	Procedure	15	4.61	Procedure	20	4.62
Remove a cemented stem	Combined	15	-	-	-	-
Implant a modular revision stem	Procedure	35	4.65	Procedure	60	4.55
Refix an ETO with cerclage wires	Procedure	10	4.70	Procedure	10	4.53
Complex total arthroplasty: knee						
Primary TKA	-	-	-	Procedure	120	4.54
Revision TKA: remove existing prosthesis	Part procedure	15	4.66	-	-	-
Revision TKA	Procedure	70	4.66	Procedure	120	4.73
Revision TKA: fixation with screws	Part procedure	15	4.64	-	-	-

(continued on next page)

Procedure (by Course Type)	Dry Bone Practical Exercises			Anatomic Specimen Laboratory		
	Type	Time	Rating	Type	Time	Rating
Periprosthetic fractures: revision						
Posterior approach to the hip	-	-	-	Approach	30	
Plate osteosynthesis of the posterior column	Procedure	-	-	Procedure	30	
Implant a revision cup with additional screw	Procedure	-	-	Procedure	70	
ETO	Procedure	-	-	Procedure	30	
Implant a modular revision stem	Procedure	70	4.82	Procedure	45	
Refix ETO with cerclage wires, GT fracture	Procedure	-	-	Procedure	45	
Periprosthetic fractures: internal fixation						
Internal fixation techniques: cables, cerclage	Tasks and test	30	4.82	Procedure	-	
Attachment plate, periprosthetic screws	Tasks and test	30	4.82	Procedure	-	
Insert a distal femoral nail	-	-	-	Procedure	30	
Interprosthetic fracture fixation	Procedure	40	4.82	Procedure	60	
Medial approach to distal femur, double-plate	-	-	-	Procedure	30	

Abbreviations: GT, greater tuberosity; THA, total hip arthroplasty; TKA, total knee arthroplasty.

procedures for joint preservation in both the hip and the knee and a new skills station for safe acetabular screw insertion. Before each event, participants are asked to complete an online self-assessment, and gaps in the competencies in performing the procedures are consistently present. These data suggest gaps exist and that the audience is highly motivated to learn in all the event types.

LESSONS LEARNED

The AO Recon Skills Laboratory integrates practical aspects into a theoretic course that existed for several years and is different to existing courses that focus only on technical expertise. The premise is to explain theoretic knowledge and philosophies to participants to further improve their performance in the operating room. To provide learners with real-time feedback, several stations contain integrated assessment tools.

For example, in reaming the acetabulum station, there are several crucial steps to be taken to prevent errors and these are highlighted in the station. It is crucial that the surgeon verifies the position of the patient and then aim for the landmarks. The model can be used in different positions and after each reaming, inclination and anteversion are measured using a laser device. This evaluation can show the learner how incorrect patient positioning may negatively affect their visual assessment of the position of the acetabulum.

Similarly, in the tibial alignment stations, a cutting guide is attached to the model and the learner must assemble and position it. As is common in practice, the learner will assess the

Table 2
Assessment tools integrated into Recon Skills Laboratory and periprosthetic fractures practical exercise

Assessment Purpose in Example	Solution	How is It Used
Assess acetabular reaming in terms of alignment for cup insertion	A laser pointer is integrated with a display screen 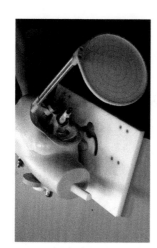	• Ream the acetabulum • Place a fixed laser source in the acetabulum and attach projector • Assess the lines and discuss the reasons for the result
Assess the alignment for a tibial cut:	A laser beam is integrated to show alignment 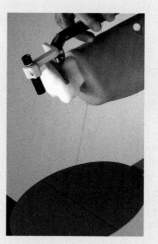	• Add the guide and adjust for the required angles until satisfied • Uncover the back plate with the laser line • Compare one line with the standard and decide why there are differences
Assess the performance of a tibial cut: provide feedback on depth and smoothness of cuts (and therefore of the cutting technique) and the amount of heat generated	A plasticized block to simulate soft tissue behind knee	• Place a new plasticized block before each cut • Perform the cut • Assess block for cuts, melting, discoloration • Discuss potential damage to soft tissues from cuts, heat, etc

- Move the "Salami" bone model for next attempt

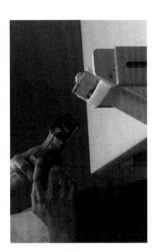

To test the strength of a series of fixation constructs: (1) cerclage wire, (2) cerclage wires, cables, plate, periprosthetic screws

Attachable balance/gauge to measure strength of construct

- Apply each technique using the simulated minimally invasive environment
  Check the strength of the construct using a weighing balance
  Discuss the constructs

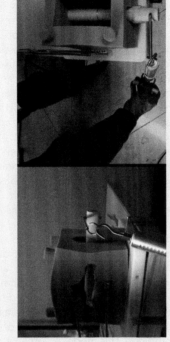

coronal alignment and posterior slope visually. The result can be judged against a laser pointing device, and assessment can reveal how well the performed alignment is compared with the optimal result. With repetition, the learner can improve his or her ability to improve the tibial cut using the immediate feedback from the laser device.

In terms of complex skills development, such as revision arthroplasty and periprosthetic fracture management, the question arose "why do we need new practical exercises in a complex course?" Precourse questionnaires revealed that surgeons from many parts of the world who are expected to practice complex arthroplasty had the theoretic knowledge but lacked the necessary experience due to low volumes. These results led to developing techniques that could be easily taught and mass-scaled at a relatively low cost, without always using expensive, difficult to obtain, cadaveric specimens. In the revision hip arthroplasty setting, models were developed to remove a well-fixed acetabular component, which is not possible in a cadaveric specimen, by manufacturing a synthetic bone model with an integrated acetabular shell. These models allowed the participant to learn how to use the tools, with the important limitation of a lack of the constraints of a soft-tissue envelope and reduced fidelity and highlights that this method of teaching has not only inherent advantages but also shortcomings. Similarly, a specific model was developed on the femoral side for removal of a well-fixed cemented stem, with the same advantages and limitations. This model

allows the teaching of an extended femoral osteotomy, as well as cement removal techniques. The same specimen can be used for simulating the insertion of a revision femoral stem; this can also be taught in a cadaveric specimen, which has the added advantage of having the constraints of a soft tissue envelope, and highlights that the various models are complementary, serving different purposes, and can be adapted to the unique needs of the learner, working within the unique conditions and regulatory environment in the geographic region where the course is taking place.

For revision knee arthroplasty, it is nearly impossible to have an anatomic specimen with a well-fixed knee replacement. A dry bone model with an integrated replica of a cemented total knee prosthesis (**Fig. 2**) and a stable holder (see **Fig. 1**) were therefore developed to enable efficient and safe use of the instruments and equipment. One advantage of using a dry bone model is that a deformity can be predefined and standardized, and this deformity can be varied based on what revision skill needs to be taught. Also, implant removal and revision techniques can be taught in one station. Finally, the model is designed to allow for some bone loss when the implant is removed, introducing the topic of bone loss management in revision total knee arthroplasty. Experience with this model emphasized the importance of having an experienced faculty member to go over the procedure in detail at a demonstration station at the beginning of the exercise, similar to an anatomic specimen station. In addition, each station requires a

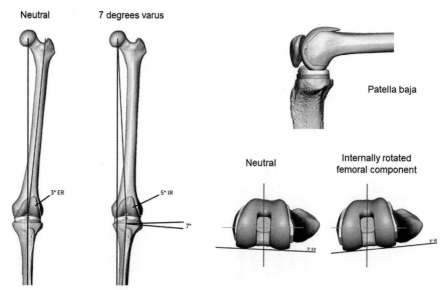

Neutral   7 degrees varus

Patella baja

Neutral   Internally rotated femoral component

Fig. 2. Specific model for knee revision arthroplasty.

skilled and experienced surgeon to support the participants. The practical stations are taught in such a way as to emphasize the importance of basic principles, avoiding focusing on the nuances of a particular implant system, with the expectation that the participant will need to adapt methods to whichever implant system is available at their respective center.

SUMMARY

Stirling's review suggested several advantages and disadvantages of the 2 simulation methods explored by AO Recon over recent years. For cadaveric models (anatomic specimens), the authors' experience supports the proposed advantages of being high fidelity and enabling instruction of both the anatomy and surgical approaches. The disadvantages include significant investments of time and the difficulty in setting these up compared with dry bone exercises, in addition to the lack of specimen uniformity and the inability to have a well-fixed prosthesis to be removed from a specimen. Although these shortcomings can be mitigated with synthetic bones, the consistent feedback is that such models lack the constraints of the soft tissue envelope, which is the primary disadvantage of these models. However, these models afford the learner the ability to operate on well-fixed implants, which is not possible in anatomic specimens. Finally, such models have the ability to integrate immediate feedback for the learner, as noted with the laser guides in the basic exercises.

According to the authors' experience with the AO Recon Skills stations, conveying the key messages is the most important aspect and is the central challenge, as opposed to learning how to use manufacturer-specific tools, as is the case with industry-led courses. The role of experienced faculty members in achieving this goal cannot be understated, as they help to transfer their knowledge to the learner, not only in a didactic manner but also using these models as an excellent practical teaching tool.

Needs Assessment in 2019
The authors conducted a global needs assessment and 319 surgeons responded to questions such as "which of the following AO Recon offerings would you participate in during the next 2 to 3 years?". Twelve percent of the surgeons reported they would attend a 2-day course without practical exercises compared with 54% and 59% who said would attend a 2-day course with practical exercises and anatomy laboratories. Sixty-six percent reported they would attend a 2.5-day course with 1 full-day anatomic specimen laboratory. The responders also have a high level of interest in online videos and in fellowships or observerships. These findings suggest that there is an ongoing need for education on primary and revision arthroplasty and related areas in many countries for both residents and qualified surgeons.

CLINICS CARE POINTS FOR EDUCATION

- Skills training in arthroplasty can focus either on "part tasks" or on full procedures.
- The curriculum committee needs to identify what learners need to be able to do effectively and safely (eg, key parts) and how to deliver an appropriate learning experience with assessment.
- Each station and practical exercise must have a clear structure with learning objectives, steps, and take-home messages.
- Faculty preparation and engagement as well as technical support and resources are required.
- Participant ratings suggest a high level of acceptance and educational value for "hands-on"—both dry bone practical exercises and anatomic specimen procedures: these can meet learner gaps.
- A combination of educational methods reinforces learning in an educational course.

ACKNOWLEDGMENTS AND FUNDING FOR THE AO RECON EXPERIENCE

Thanks to all the surgeon faculty who designed the stations and practical exercises and to all the faculty and participants who tested and implemented these and provided feedback. Thanks also to the Curriculum taskforces members Dr Robert Hube, Dr Michael Huo, and all AO Recon faculty who helped; the AO Recon Education Forum (chairperson Carsten Perka and all members); the AO Recon team; the AO Education Institute curriculum development, video, and publishing teams; Felix Burr and Robert Ferus (Synbone); Peter Sauter (Fabritastika); Barbara Goldenberger (DePuy Synthes); and Cynthia Stampfli. We also thank DePuy Synthes for an educational grant that provided funding for the development and their support in implementation during the courses.

DISCLOSURE

The authors have nothing to disclose.

REFERENCES

1. Walter AJ. Surgical education for the twenty-first century: beyond the apprentice model. Obstet Gynecol Clin North Am 2006;33(2):233–6, vii.
2. Osmanski-Zenk K, Finze S, Lenz R, et al. Influence of training of orthopaedic surgeons on clinical outcome after total hip arthroplasty in a high volume endoprosthetic centre. Z Orthop Unfall 2019; 157(1):48–53.
3. Storey R, Frampton C, Kieser D, et al. Does orthopaedic training compromise the outcome in knee joint arthroplasty? J Surg Educ 2018;75(5):1292–8.
4. Bell RH Jr, Biester TW, Tabuenca A, et al. Operative experience of residents in US general surgery programs: a gap between expectation and experience. Ann Surg 2009;249(5):719–24.
5. Kim SC, Fisher JG, Delman KA, et al. Cadaver-based simulation increases resident confidence, initial exposure to fundamental techniques, and may augment operative autonomy. J Surg Educ 2016;73(6):e33–41.
6. The Impact of EWTD on Delivery of Surgical Services: A Consensus Statement. Association of Surgeons of Great Britain and Ireland. 2008. Available at: https://www.asgbi.org.uk/publications/working-time-regulations. Accessed July 5, 2020.
7. Philibert I, Friedmann P, Williams WT. New requirements for resident duty hours. JAMA 2002;288(9): 1112–4.
8. Reidy MJ, Faulkner A, Shitole B, et al. Do trainee surgeons have an adverse effect on the outcome after total hip arthroplasty?: a ten-year review. Bone Joint J 2016;98-b(3):301–6.
9. Moran M, Yap SL, Walmsley P, et al. Clinical and radiologic outcome of total hip arthroplasty performed by trainee compared with consultant orthopedic surgeons. J Arthroplasty 2004;19(7):853–7.
10. Palan J, Gulati A, Andrew JG, et al. The trainer, the trainee and the surgeons' assistant: clinical outcomes following total hip replacement. J Bone Joint Surg Br 2009;91(7):928–34.
11. Kazarian GS, Lawrie CM, Barrack TN, et al. The impact of surgeon volume and training status on implant alignment in total knee arthroplasty. J Bone Joint Surg Am 2019;101(19):1713–23.
12. Holt G, Nunn T, Gregori A. Ethical dilemmas in orthopaedic surgical training. J Bone Joint Surg Am 2008;90(12):2798–803.
13. Nzeako O, Back D. Learning Curves in Arthroplasty in Orthopedic Trainees. J Surg Educ 2016;73(4): 689–93.
14. Stirling ER, Lewis TL, Ferran NA. Surgical skills simulation in trauma and orthopaedic training. J Orthop Surg Res 2014;9:126.
15. Gaba DM. The future vision of simulation in health care. Qual Saf Health Care 2004;13(Suppl 1):i2–10.
16. Anastakis DJ, Regehr G, Reznick RK, et al. Assessment of technical skills transfer from the bench training model to the human model. Am J Surg 1999;177(2):167–70.
17. Rinaldo S. W5 probes the shadowy world of a body broker dealing in human remains 2019. Available at: https://www.ctvnews.ca/w5/w5-probes-the-shadowy-world-of-a-body-broker-dealing-in-human-remains-1.4297489. Accessed July 14, 2020.
18. Bergeson RK, Schwend RM, DeLucia T, et al. How accurately do novice surgeons place thoracic pedicle screws with the free hand technique? Spine (Phila Pa 1976) 2008;33(15):E501–7.
19. Bell CD, O'Sullivan JG, Ostervoss TE, et al. Surgical simulation maximizing the use of fresh-frozen cadaveric specimens: examination of tissue integrity using ultrasound. J Grad Med Educ 2020; 12(3):329–34.
20. Sonnadara RR, Van Vliet A, Safir O, et al. Orthopedic boot camp: examining the effectiveness of an intensive surgical skills course. Surgery 2011;149(6):745–9.
21. Hausmann JT. Sawbones in biomechanical settings - a review. Osteosynthesis and Trauma Care 2006; 14(04):259–64. Available at: HYPERLINK "https://nam03.safelinks.protection.outlook.com/?url=https%3A%2F%2Fwww.thieme-connect.de%2Fproducts%2Fejournals%2Fabstract%2F10.1055%2Fs-2006-942333&data=02%7C01%7CJ.Surendrakumar%40elsevier.com%7C1623717c3772479526b508d86bc8acdf%7C9274ee3f94254109a27f9fb15c10675d%7C0%7C0%7C637377857730435669&sdata=RTvFofJpA7aTk2zGe33zBHV%2F6SQ8T51VmnvPbLQTqZA%3D&reserved=0" Available at: https://www.thieme-connect.de/products/ejournals/abstract/10.1055/s-2006-942333.
22. Lewis TL, Vohra RS. Smartphones make smarter surgeons. Br J Surg 2014;101(4):296–7.
23. Kahol K, Vankipuram M, Smith ML. Cognitive simulators for medical education and training. J Biomed Inform 2009;42(4):593–604.
24. Kohls-Gatzoulis JA, Regehr G, Hutchison C. Teaching cognitive skills improves learning in surgical skills courses: a blinded, prospective, randomized study. Can J Surg 2004;47(4):277–83.
25. Aïm F, Lonjon G, Hannouche D, et al. Effectiveness of virtual reality training in orthopaedic surgery. Arthroscopy 2016;32(1):224–32.
26. Pedowitz RA, Esch J, Snyder S. Evaluation of a virtual reality simulator for arthroscopy skills development. Arthroscopy 2002;18(6):E29.

27. Gomoll AH, O'Toole RV, Czarnecki J, et al. Surgical experience correlates with performance on a virtual reality simulator for shoulder arthroscopy. Am J Sports Med 2007;35(6):883–8.

28. McCarthy AD, Moody L, Waterworth AR, et al. Passive haptics in a knee arthroscopy simulator: is it valid for core skills training? Clin Orthop Relat Res 2006;442:13–20.

29. Kalun P, Wagner N, Yan J, et al. Surgical simulation training in orthopedics: current insights. Adv Med Educ Pract 2018;9:125–31.

30. Lohre R, Bois AJ, Athwal GS, et al, on behalf of the Canadian S, Elbow Society. Improved complex skill acquisition by immersive virtual reality training: a randomized controlled trial. J Bone Joint Surg Am 2020;102(6):e26.

Augmented Reality in Orthopedic Practice and Education

Timothy C. Keating, MD[a],*, Joshua J. Jacobs, MD[b]

KEYWORDS

- Augmented reality • Mixed reality • Total knee arthroplasty • Total hip arthroplasty
- Computer-assisted surgery • Navigation • Head-mounted display

KEY POINTS

- The tracking functionality, system control software, and a human-machine interface of traditional surgical navigation may be consolidated to new augmented reality (AR) headsets.
- AR technology has special promise for advancing hip and knee arthroplasty navigation.
- AR also has the potential to accelerate and improve surgical education.

INTRODUCTION TO AUGMENTED REALITY

Augmented reality (AR) technology is used to enhance a user's perception and interaction with the natural world through the superimposition of digital information on physical images.[1,2] The user experience of AR exists on the reality-virtuality continuum described by Milgram in 1994 (Fig. 1) that describes the overlap of the physical world and a digital world.[3] Unlike immersive virtual reality (VR) that creates a total virtual experience, augmented, or mixed reality (AR/MR) encompasses the middle of the reality-virtuality continuum and allows for continued interaction with the real world.[2,4]

The first AR device was a headset created by Sutherland in 1968 that had to be mounted to the ceiling because of the weight of the device.[5] This device was the first to create an optical see-through display using 2 cathode-ray tubes that created a digital overlay.[6] This is contrasted with the video see-through capabilities of some systems where the real and digital worlds are combined and displayed on a standard video monitor.[2,7] The development of AR in recent decades has been funded by the US National Aeronautics and Space Administration (NASA) and other government agencies to develop training simulators for space exploration and aircraft navigation.[8] The heads-up display of an airplane cockpit (Fig. 2A) is 1 example of an optical see-through device that was developed to provide pilots with information like altitude, speed, horizon, and prompts that make up a ground collision avoidance system. US Air Force pilots now benefit from the same augmented flying experience with next-generation optical see-through technology incorporated into small helmet-mounted displays (Fig. 2B).[9]

AR headsets have recently become available direct to consumers with applications typically aimed at enhancing smartphone interconnectedness (eg, Google Glass [Google, Mountain View, California]), which was released to the public in 2014.[10] Equipped with a single standard definition (SD) camera and simple holographic projection system, Google Glass connects to enabled devices and allows users to view emails and messages, receive turn-by-turn navigation, or even read the New York Times.[11] (Fig. 3A). Alternatively, some AR devices are designed specifically for enterprise

[a] Department of Orthopedic Surgery, Rush University Medical Center, 1611 West Harrison Street, Suite 301, Chicago, IL 60612, USA; [b] Department of Orthopedic Surgery, Rush University Medical Center, 1611 West Harrison Street, Suite 201, Chicago, IL 60612, USA
* Corresponding author.
E-mail address: timothy_c_keating@rush.edu

Orthop Clin N Am 52 (2021) 15–26
https://doi.org/10.1016/j.ocl.2020.08.002

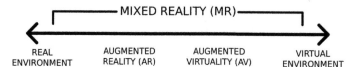

Fig. 1. The reality-virtuality continuum. First defined by Milgram in 1994,[3] mixed reality encompasses the overlap of the real and digital worlds, with AR based predominantly on real-world images supplemented with digital overlay. AR navigation in surgery allows an unobstructed view of the surgical field with an overlay of supplemental information. (*From* Milgram, Paul & Kishino, Fumio. A Taxonomy of Mixed Reality Visual Displays vol. E77-D, no. 12. 1321-1329. IEICE Trans. Information Systems. Copyright © 2016 IEICE. Used with permission.)

applications. The Hololens 2 (Microsoft Corporation, Redmond, Washington), released in 2019, is 1 example of a highly equipped AR headset sporting 5 high-definition (HD) optical cameras, a binocular, eye-tracking, display capable of generating holograms with meaningful position and orientation in the real world, enterprise-grade iris recognition security, and sensors to detect simultaneous hand position for interactive gestures (Fig. 3B).[12] AR headsets have become increasingly sophisticated with advances in the individual technologies that provide their displays, power, wireless connectivity, computing, and sensing capabilities.

AUGMENTED REALITY NAVIGATION IN COMPUTER-ASSISTED SURGERY

Within health care, AR has proven to be a useful adjunct to computer-assisted surgery (CAS), which aims to improve patient outcomes through increased surgical precision and less invasive surgery.[13] At the core of CAS is surgical navigation enabled by tracking functionality, system control software, and a human-machine interface. In a standard surgical navigation system, tracking functionality utilizing fiducial markers within the sterile field to reference surgical anatomy and surgical instruments within the same Cartesian coordinate system.[14] Fiducial markers are most commonly tracked using cameras off the sterile field that function within the infrared wavelength, with markers considered active if they emit infrared light and passive if they only reflect infrared light.[15] AR navigation instead uses a standard red-green-blue (RGB) camera to track markers within the sterile field (eg, a standard AR fiducial marker) (Fig. 4A), Quick Response (QR) codes (Fig. 4B), or any other predetermined pattern or object through pattern or object-recognition software.[2] The video input in AR navigation applications can be provided by cameras on an AR headset, reducing line-of-sight issues and eliminating the setup of off-field cameras.

System control software is the collective software and hardware necessary to process the input from tracked markers to generate the position and orientation of a tracked object. In standard navigation, input from cameras away from the sterile field is processed with stand-alone computer hardware and software.[1] AR headsets are equipped with computers that

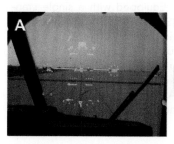
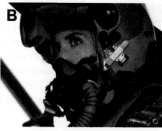

Fig. 2. Optical see-through displays in aviation. (*A*): A Lockheed C-130 Hercules military jet equipped with an optical see-through device to display flight information.[73] Recent optical display technology has allowed these systems to be scaled down to helmet- and headset-mounted technology. In Fig. 2B, a US Air Force fighter pilot is equipped with a helmet-mounted optical see-through device over her right eye that displays similar flight information.[9] Permissions: Fig. 2A labeled for reuse according to Creative Commons Attribution 2.0 Generic License, Fig. 2B labeled for reuse as part of the Public Domain according to Department of Defense Instruction 5410.20, image labeled and cropped to emphasize the subject. *Disclaimer: The appearance of U.S. Department of Defense (DoD) visual information does not imply or constitute DoD endorsement.* ([A] *From* Lappin T. C-130 jet: Co-pilot's head-up display panel. November 2004; with permission.; and [B] *Courtesy of* Staff Sgt. Samantha Mathison, Fort Worth, Texas.)

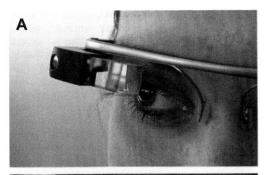

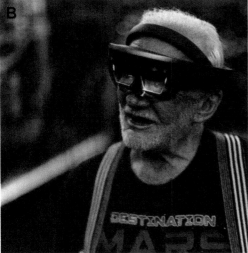

Fig. 3. Spectrum of AR headsets. (*A*): Google Glass, released to the public in 2014, has a small optical see-through lens that projects a digital image onto the user's retina to create a hologram. The hologram is static in relation to the headset, which connects to a smartphone or other enabled device through short-range wireless technology.[10] (*B*): Apollo 11 astronaut Buzz Aldrin trials the Hololens at a Kennedy Space Center exhibit where visitors are guided through imagery captured by NASA's Mars rover, Curiosity, by a holographic Buzz Aldrin.[74] Permissions: Fig. 3A labeled for reuse according to Creative Commons Attribution 2.0 Generic License, Fig. 3B cropped to emphasize the subject, labeled for reuse as part of the public domain as property of NASA. (*From* Google "Project Glass" replaces the smartphone with glasses. PCMAG. https://www.pcmag.com/archive/google-project-glass-replaces-the-smartphone-with-glasses-296284. Accessed July 24, 2020 and Babir N. Apollo 11 astronaut Buzz Aldrin tries out Microsoft HoloLens mixed reality headset. September 2016. https://www.flickr.com/photos/nasakennedy/29794543715/. Accessed July 24, 2020.)

can process input to a degree that eliminates the need for an off-field stand-alone computer. AR technology must process input to an additional degree, calculating the pose of the headset in relation to the marker in order to later display digital images with a meaningful position and orientation in the real world.[16]

Navigation information is delivered to the surgeon through a human-machine interface, which in a conventional system comprises a video monitor that requires the surgeon to divert his or her attention from the operative field. An AR system with an optical see-through equipped headset allows navigation information to appear overlaid on real objects in the operative field so that a surgeon can focus his or her attention on the patient and enjoy more natural navigation prompts.[17,18] Aside from wearable headsets, other display options include transparent screens over the operative field, in-field tablets with video see-through capability, or projector-based systems that project virtual images directly on real objects.[13]

GENERAL ORTHOPEDIC APPLICATIONS OF AUGMENTED REALITY

The utility of AR navigation was first demonstrated in cardiothoracic surgery using MRI-based guidance for endovascular procedures on a beating heart[19] and laparoscopic surgery using AR overlay of important anatomic structures during laparoscopic cholecystectomy.[20] Since then, applications have expanded to most surgical fields including orthopedic surgery.[1] Computer-assisted orthopedic surgery, in general, has experienced a robust and diverse evolution since its conception in the 1980s.[21] Technological advance has encompassed surgical education, planning, navigation, robotic assistance, and now AR navigation.[22]

In orthopedic trauma, preclinical applications have shown promising results in guidance for interlocking screws in nails, guide-wire placement in dynamic hip screws, and osteosynthesis of pelvic fractures.[23–27] Londei and colleagues[24] showed that a C-arm combined with a tracking camera allowed users to successfully place distal interlocking screws in a femoral intramedullary nail 93% of the time, which greatly reduces the burden of ionizing radiation typically required to place distal interlocking screws. Dynamic hip screw stabilization for extracapsular hip fractures relies on accurate guidewire placement and has also been an area of interest for AR guidance.[25] Utilizing orthogonal cameras and tracked instruments, van Duren and colleagues developed a system capable of overlaying digital instrument position and orientation on fluoroscopic images obtained during guidewire placement. This system enabled a real-time display of tip-apex

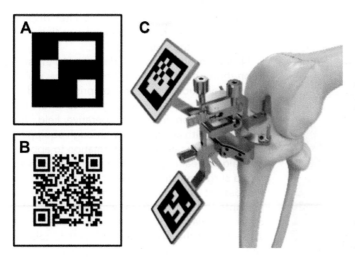

Fig. 4. 2-dimensional markers for 3-dimensional registration in AR. AR systems are capable of tracking several different types of markers, including (*A*), a standard AR marker, (*B*) a QR code, or any other recognizable pattern. Once localized, the orientation of these markers is calculated based on their appearance and a unique coordinate system is assigned. 4C demonstrates a clinical example of 2-dimensional markers affixed to a proprietary tibial cutting guide used in AR navigation. The pictured system was the first used in a live surgery using AR navigation for TKA in 2020. ([*C*] *Courtesy of* Pixee Medical, Besançon, France; with permission.)

distance for the guidewire that was accurate within 2 mm of error after calibration.[25] Osteosynthesis of complex pelvic fractures has also been investigated, as a pilot study by Befrui and colleagues[27] in 2018 showed that AR navigation enabled by hybrid cone-beam C-arm fluoroscopy and a standard RGB camera decreased operative time and radiation dose compared with standard methods of screw placement.

Hand surgery has benefited from AR through wrist arthroscopy navigation, which allowed a digital overlay of the position and orientation of the wrist arthroscope on a fluoroscopic image of the wrist during scope insertion surgery.[28] Finally, spine surgery, and specifically pedicle screw insertion, has already seen multiple applications of AR navigation.[29,30] In 2018, a new system enabled precise placement of thoracolumbar pedicle screws through registration of preoperative imaging and planning with an intraoperative computed tomography (CT) scan.[31] During the procedure, digital overlay from 4 tracking cameras displayed real-time location of instrumentation in relation to patient anatomy to guide pedicle screw insertion. The authors of this study demonstrated that pedicle screws were placed inside the pedicle 100% of the time, with a deviation of 2.2 mm plus or minus 1.3 mm from the planned path.[31] The first-ever live surgery with a similar system of AR navigation for pedicle screw placement in a minimally invasive posterior spinal fusion was recently performed at the authors' institution with an encouraging early clinical result.[32]

This article focuses on the great potential for AR navigation in total knee arthroplasty (TKA) and total hip arthroplasty (THA). A medical subject heading (MeSH) search of the MEDLINE Pubmed library was conducted using the phrase "(mixed OR augmented) reality (hip OR knee)."[33] The inclusion criteria for the search targeted articles that reported developing a preclinical or clinical application of AR in TKA and THA, as well as the topic of TKA and THA education and professional development. In total, 46 items were available for review, five of which were suitable for inclusion for TKA, 4 articles for THA, and 5 articles for professional development and education relating to arthroplasty.

AUGMENTED REALITY APPLICATIONS IN ARTHROPLASTY
Total Knee Arthroplasty

AR technology has special promise for hip and knee arthroplasty. The primary objectives of TKA are maximizing implant function and longevity through restoring a natural limb alignment, implanting components perpendicular to the limb mechanical axis, and ensuring appropriate soft tissue balance through balanced extension and flexion gaps.[34,35] These goals have historically been achieved with manual instrumentation, but in recent years various technologies have been incorporated in an effort to increase surgical precision. Guiding tibial alignment has been accomplished through directly instrumenting the intramedullary canal of the tibia, or aligning extramedullary guides to anatomic landmarks.[36] Recent navigation technology guides tibial resection according to the mechanical axis through referencing similar anatomic landmarks in an imageless system, or a combination of anatomic landmarks and intraoperative registering of preoperative 3-dimensional imaging in an image-based system.[37] Femoral alignment in navigated TKA typically tracks a dynamic movement of the femur during hip circumduction to locate the hip center and thus the mechanical axis of the femur.[38]

AR has been recently introduced to TKA as a means to facilitate navigation. Pokhrel and colleagues[39] developed a system to facilitate the real-time superimposition of a preoperative CT scan on the surgical field for feedback and optimization of planned bone resection. Their system relies on an iterative closest point (ICP) algorithm that matches points on the surface of the 3D preoperative CT scans to points on video images of the same bony anatomy obtained intraoperatively. After referencing, the desired bony resection is calculated based on the preoperative plan and is updated in real time to reflect what bone still has to be resected using a heat map with different colors corresponding to remaining resection depth. That image is displayed onto a transparent screen over the surgical field to create the AR experience for the surgeon. The results of their preclinical trials of this technology show a standard error of bone resection of between 0.40 and 0.55 mm. One potential downside of this technology is that the complex data processing results in a display frame rate between 12 to 13 frames per second, which would appear to lag compared with the 30 frames per second rate of standard high definition video.[40]

Wang and colleagues[41] also developed an AR application to assist visualization in TKA, this time built on the Microsoft Hololens (Microsoft Corporation). Their system also registers a preoperative CT to in-field markers using a tracked stylus, collecting data points known as a point cloud,[41] which are then matched to the preoperative CT with an ICP algorithm similar to that described by Pokhrel and colleagues.[39] Once registered, the Hololens projects the 3-dimensional model from the preoperative CT on real patient anatomy to guide resection. The results of this investigation were promising in regards to precision, as the root mean square error of point cloud registration was 1.08 mm for the femoral model and 1.78 mm for the tibial model. With this registration, the actual holographic overlay was within 2.5 mm of the models, which they deemed within a reasonable margin of error.[41] One of the potential advantages of this preclinical study is the incorporation of an AR headset, although this system still employs the use of an off-field depth camera to assist in headset localization. Future wearable devices would ideally have an improved capacity for self-localization and calibration for accurate hologram overlay. Another potential limitation of the described system is the overlay accuracy of the hologram at 2.5 mm, which may not be acceptable for an application guiding bony cuts near at-risk anatomic structures.

Daniel and Ramos in 2016 took a different approach to an AR application for TKA.[42] Instead of focusing on the registration of preoperative imaging, their study utilized imageless registration with 2-dimensional markers equivalent to those used in other AR applications (see Fig. 4A). With 1 marker attached to the tibia and another to the femur, knee flexion and extension define 6° of freedom of knee articulation. Their investigation also proposed the concept of using virtual models of available tibial and femoral components in calculations to optimize component position within the bounds of knee motion to yield balanced tibiofemoral gaps. One of the potential drawbacks of their developed system is that the accuracy is highly dependent on how close the markers are to each other, with error increasing exponentially as the markers are farther apart. At 20 cm of marker separation, the absolute error of virtual model projection was only 0.8 mm but increased to about 4 mm of error at 30 cm of separation.[42] This error will have to be optimized before a true clinical application while still keeping the markers from interfering with the surgical field. Imageless navigation could result in cost savings, and, in the case of systems requiring a preoperative CT, radiation saving. Another potential benefit of this approach is the intraoperative time savings of avoiding the point cloud registration process. The authors propose the use of additional markers to increase system precision and the use of infrared markers to eliminate the variability associated with changing light conditions in the operating room as subjects of future studies.[42]

The final preclinical knee study revealed by the authors' literature search is a smartphone application named "AR-knee" by Tsukada and colleagues[43] to navigate the tibial cut in TKA. Instead of using an optical see-through screen such as a transparent display over the field[39] or a head-mounted display (HMD),[41] the application uses the camera and display of a smartphone to create video see-through AR. Their system works by placing a smartphone into a sealed, sterile case to be brought into the operative field in a way that allows for continued interaction with the smartphone touchscreen. Using a tracked pointer, 7 tibial landmarks are registered to a marker attached to the tibia. Landmarks include the medial malleolus, lateral malleolus, the center of the tibial plateau, the center of the posterior cruciate ligament insertion on the tibia, the medial border of the patellar tendon insertion, the center of the medial plateau, and the center of the lateral plateau.[43] By registering these anatomic points, a tibial coordinate system is established consisting of the longitudinal axis of the tibia in the coronal plane, the tibial slope in the sagittal plane, and the anteroposterior axis of the tibia in the axial plane. Displaying these virtual axes on the tibia allows the surgeon to visually align the tibial cutting guide before making the tibial cut. Tibial alignment is checked by placing a third marker on the cut surface of the tibia and displaying the orientation of that marker within the tibial coordinate system. Tsukada and colleagues tested their system in a Sawbones model (Sawbones USA, Vashon Island, Washington) executing tibial resections in 10 instances and confirming the alignment with CT scans. They found the varus/valgus and posterior slope of the tibial resection to be within 1° of the plan, and the axial alignment of the tibial resection to be within 2°, none of which were significantly different ($P > .05$) from the plan. This system overall demonstrated excellent precision compared with other reported systems[44] and is a promising technology. Although using the surgeon's personal smartphone is an innovative cost-saving measure, relying on a specialized smartphone case to maintain sterility may complicate reprocessing and ultimately increase costs compared with an AR headset system.

Although the aforementioned studies have evaluated AR in preclinical studies for navigating TKA, only recently has this technology made its debut in actual clinical use.[45] In 2020, the first TKA using AR technology was performed in Paris.[46] This system uses 2-dimensional trackers affixed to novel TKA instrumentation shown in Fig. 4C.[47] This system is based on commercially available AR glasses,[48] and uses marker-based anatomic registration to establish tibial and femoral alignment. During surgery, the user receives holographic guidance indicating a planned tibial and femoral resection angle and depth. Published preclinical and clinical studies will be needed to evaluate the accuracy and precision of the system, but preliminary capabilities alone are promising. Like other systems with simple marker navigation, this system has the advantage of being imageless and does not consume disposables. As the first stand-alone AR headset system, this setup is an excellent example of the true potential for portable, cost-effective AR navigation in TKA.

A second application of AR in TKA was even more recently announced to have been granted US Food and Drug Administration clearance for use in the United States.[49] This technology also appears to be based on off-the-shelf AR glasses, although a novel tracking method has been introduced that uses disposable Bluetooth-enabled infrared trackers. Although the cost of consumable technology appears to be an early disadvantage of this type of system, the clinical utility and precision have yet to be published and may justify the cost. The coming years are likely to see a rapid expansion of clinical applications for AR in the world of TKA.

Augmented Reality in Total Hip Arthroplasty

Accurate component position in THA is of utmost importance in order to restore native biomechanics and reduce the risk of leg-length inequality, accelerated component wear, impingement, and dislocation.[50] Although the true safe zone for acetabular cup position may be a moving target based on many factors, the ability to reliably hit a certain position target is also a necessity.[50,51] Numerous computer-assisted applications for acetabular cup navigation have been developed in recent years that utilize either an image-based or imageless registration process to determine and display the position of the acetabular cup in relation to the patient's pelvis.[14] Given the same limitations of traditional navigation as described previously for TKA (ie, setup, line-of-sight issues with marker tracking, and diverting surgeon attention), AR has a great potential to improve THA.

In 2008 Fotouhi and colleagues[52] introduced an AR navigation system for cup placement in THA. They found available image-based navigation systems to be unsatisfactory because of the added cost and radiation exposure of a preoperative CT, and the added intraoperative time required for registration. Additionally, they found that intraoperative fluoroscopic guidance often used in anterior approach THA required the surgeon to determine the 3-dimensional pose of the cup from a 2-dimensional image, which is prone to error.[52] In light of existing shortcomings, their system uses AR to create a reliable, reproducible system for cup implantation that reduces radiation exposure and works naturally into a surgical workflow. Their system relies on a custom configuration of C-arm fitted with a camera that is equipped with RGB and depth functionality (RBG-D). Much like a standard surgical workflow, the surgeon obtains an anteroposterior (AP) pelvis fluoroscopic view in order to align the detector with the anterior pelvic plane (APP) after reaming the acetabulum. The surgeon then positions a virtual cup at the correct translation on the AP image, opting for a preset anteversion and inclination. Because the field of view of the RGB-D camera and C-arm are calibrated prior to the procedure, placing the virtual cup at a certain 2-dimensional coordinate within the AP pelvis allows the system to compute and anticipate the ideal position of the inserter handle rigidly attached to the cup. During cup implantation, the RGB-D camera tracks the location and orientation of the cup handle and produces an AR image of 2 orthogonal planes to guide cup position. Viewing these 2 planes simultaneously allows the surgeon to make precise adjustments to the cup orientation. The precision of this system in a simulated preclinical study demonstrated a standard error of 1.9 mm of translation, 1.1° of abduction, and 0.53° of anteversion, which is comparable to if not more accurate than conventional systems.[52,53] The same institution later tested this AR-based system compared to standard fluoroscopy with 8 senior resident participants.[54] Accuracy of cup implantation significantly favored the AR application compared with standard fluoroscopy (P<.05) in inclination and anteversion, while the precision of the AR-based system was also significantly higher for cup anteversion. Secondary outcomes of the study showed that the AR-based method took less time and demonstrated a decreased workload based on a validated assessment of usability, the Surgical Task Load Index.[54,55] This demonstration of AR-based technology in THA promises a bright future for AR with the possibility of improving patient outcomes.

The same team that produced the AR-Knee application, Tsukada and colleagues,[43,56] has also worked on bringing AR to THA. In a pilot study, a sterile guide that rests over the bilateral anterior superior iliac spines (ASIS) and pubic tubercle introduced a 2-dimensional AR marker to register the anterior pelvic plane (APP). Using the system as a measurement tool in a preclinical study, the position of a cup implanted with standard instrumentation was registered to a 2-dimensional AR marker by reattaching the cup inserter and aligning a virtual cup inserter in a video see-through AR program. These intraoperative measurements were validated on a postoperative CT scan. Compared with postoperative CT, the AR system had an absolute error and standard deviation of 2.1°plus or minus 1.5° for measuring inclination and 2.7° plus or minus 1.7° for measuring anteversion.[56] There was no difference in the ability of the AR technology to measure inclination compared with the intraoperative goniometer, but it was significantly better at predicting anteversion (P<.0001).

After a promising pilot study, this system was later used in a randomized clinical trial as intraoperative navigation.[57] Prior to surgical positioning, the APP was registered to an interosseous 2-dimensional AR marker by simultaneously resting markers on the bilateral ASIS and pubic tubercle in the supine position.[57] The patient was then put in the lateral decubitus position, prepared, and draped in a standard fashion incorporating the intraosseous AR marker into the field to maintain APP referencing. The surgeon's smartphone was placed in a special sterile sleeve for use on the sterile field. Patients were randomized to receive cup implantation with smartphone AR navigation, or standard implantation with a freehand mechanical alignment guide. At 3 months postoperatively, a CT scan was obtained, and inclination and anteversion were calculated based on the radiographic method.[57,58] Compared with the AR-navigated values of inclination and anteversion, postoperative CT showed a mean absolute difference of 1.9° plus or minus 1.3° of inclination and 2.8° plus or minus 2.2° of anteversion. Although the conventional instrumentation group was significantly less accurate in executing desired inclination (mean absolute error 3.4° plus or minus 2.6°, P=.02), the study group concluded that this was likely not a clinically significant difference. Further studies should determine whether this difference is only clinically insignificant when an experienced surgeon is the test subject, as it could be an important technology for trainees.

Augmented Reality in Arthroplasty Education and Professional Development

Beyond a purely clinical application of AR in arthroplasty is the great potential to accelerate and improve surgical education. Training to become an expert surgeon requires understanding complex physiologic systems, developing adaptive expertise in responding to all surgical possibilities, and learning how to collaborate within a multidisciplinary medical team.[59] The total immersive environment of a VR headset has gained increasing recognition for its use as a surgical training tool, but AR may offer some distinct advantages.[59–61] First, because AR allows continued interaction with the real environment, surgical training can take place with real tools in actual or simulated surgery to maximize the authenticity of the learning environment. Second, with capabilities such as overlaying the location of important anatomic structures and dangers on the surgical field, a deeper understanding of surgical anatomy along with increased safety is achieved. Third, AR experiences allow for remote observation and interaction with surgical mentors and automated guidance without a mentor.[59] Ponce and colleagues[62] described and trialed virtual interactive presence in a shoulder arthroscopy application that allowed an attending surgeon in a nearby room to interact with the resident through audio and a virtual overlay on the arthroscopy tower monitor for pointing and demonstrating maneuvers. Applying this technology to shoulder arthroscopy was found to be safe, efficient, and effective as a teaching tool.[62]

Surgical training for acetabular cup placement in THA has been an educational focus of AR applications.[63–65] In 2018 Condino and colleagues[64] developed a surgical simulator for cup placement in THA based on the Microsoft Hololens. Their system uses a pelvic model and gives the user the capability to scroll through 3-dimensional imaging and overlay the imaging on the pelvic model based on a built-in 2-dimensional marker. Available imaging modes include bony and soft tissue anatomy and the preoperative plan for THA. The accuracy of the imaging overlay was not tested objectively, but subjective evaluation of the video, audio, interaction, and ergonomics showed favorable preliminary results.[64,65] This system would benefit from an objective evaluation of overlay accuracy and application to specific surgical training.

Logishetty and colleagues[63] continued the application of HMD to hip arthroplasty. Their study randomized 24 medical students with no prior experience in hip arthroplasty to undergo 4 training sessions in acetabular cup placement with either holographic guidance from a Hololens headset or one-on-one instruction from an arthroplasty surgeon. In a final evaluation of simulated acetabular cup placement, both groups improved significantly from their baseline test and ended up equally accurate in acetabular cup placement.[63] This study suggests that automated AR guidance may approach the utility of one-on-one coaching for complex tasks.

The concept of telepresence and telemonitoring during surgery has been explored by other authors as a powerful tool not just for teaching new surgeons, but for the professional development of established surgeons.[4,66] These capabilities employ the video recording, audio, and wireless data transmission capabilities of an AR headset to conference with a surgeon in another location.[59] This technology would make telementoring of surgeons in remote areas possible during routine professional development or in cases of virtual support for difficult cases.[4]

AR also has the potential to advance surgical planning, as preoperative imaging can be displayed in 3 dimensions as a hologram that can be manipulated alongside models of implants. This technology allows for applications such as planning difficult cases on an individual basis or routinely planning implant choice and placement in arthroplasty based on 3-dimensional rather than 2-dimensional fit. For instance, certain proximal femoral morphologies may be better visualized and manipulated in 3 dimensions when planning for the ideal fit of a femoral component in THA, as some anatomic variants may be more prone to intraoperative fracture with certain stem types.[67] Another intraoperative use of AR is putting additional information at a surgeon's fingertips while maintaining sterility. Through interactive commands, an AR headset or touchscreen could be used to access information such as preoperative plans, patient medical records, additional imaging, or technical specifications of surgical implants. The use of an AR headset to access a preoperative plan intraoperatively during shoulder arthroplasty was first carried out in 2020,[68] and additional applications of these already-available technologies will certainly follow suit in the near future.

SUMMARY

The rapid expansion of AR technology has allowed an increasing number of applications in orthopedic surgery. In TKA, tibial component alignment with the mechanical axis of the tibia has been the main application AR navigation. Although initial applications utilized 3-dimensional registration to navigate a planned tibial cut,[39,41] more recent applications have utilized imageless, marker-based navigation.[42,43,47] Other investigations of imageless navigation in TKA have shown it to be accurate, cost-effective, and radiation-saving.[37] Femoral mechanical alignment based on tracking a femoral marker during hip circumduction is currently the favored method of acquiring the hip center in imageless navigation and has been adopted by available AR navigation systems.[45,69] The incorporation of trackable markers into existing instrumentation is a thoughtful step toward eliminating the time and associated risks of installing transosseous markers as required in some navigation systems.[47,70] In addition to establishing mechanical alignment in TKA, AR navigation also has the tracking and computing capabilities to offer predictive ligament balancing and component sizing. This capability will have to be developed alongside existing technology in order to secure a definite advantage over conventional TKA instrumentation and has the potential to increase patient satisfaction and function through promoting optimal knee kinematics.[71]

Total hip arthroplasty has also benefited from early AR applications that have focused on cup position. One deficiency thus far in applying AR to THA is the exclusion of femoral component navigation, which should be possible even in an imageless application with the tracking and computational functionality of available AR headsets. Further studies in AR THA applications should continue to refine the technology and compare its accuracy and surgical experience with existing navigation systems.

AR technology likely represents the future of surgical navigation. The recent development of compact, high-definition sensors and microprocessors has already equipped AR headsets with the necessary tools to absorb the cumbersome off-field tracking and display functionality of current navigation systems. Once ported to wearable AR technology, a complete surgical navigation system will be convenient enough to carry between multiple operating locations and require minimal setup and ancillary help. Most importantly, this technology promises an augmented surgical experience to promote efficient and effective surgery. AR applications have already begun to benefit from crossover from the disciplines of machine learning and artificial intelligence to improve marker-based and markerless tracking,[72] and further developments in these fields will continue to improve surgical precision. In addition, the increasing use of robotics in orthopedic surgery predicts a synergistic future with AR that will further advance the field. Although AR applications in arthroplasty may be in their infancy, they will likely mature over the next few years to become major tools in the family of available orthopedic technologies.

CLINICS CARE POINTS

- AR is a technology that enables the overlay of digital information on objects in the real world via a head-mounted display, transparent screen, or a video monitor. Existing applications in orthopedic surgery span the disciplines of trauma, hand, spine, and total joint surgery.
- Preclinical applications dedicated to acetabular cup placement in THA and tibial component alignment in TKA demonstrate accuracy equivalent to available navigation systems. Clinical applications have become available within the last year and will require published verifications alongside other available systems to promote widespread use. The future of navigation in arthroplasty will likely be dominated by wearable technology that can combine the tracking, computation, and display technology of traditional navigation into a compact and cost-effective platform.

DISCLOSURE

Neither author has anything to disclose in relation to this review, and no funding was received.

REFERENCES

1. Chytas D, Malahias M-A, Nikolaou VS. Augmented reality in orthopedics: current state and future directions. Front Surg 2019;6:38.
2. Carmigniani J, Furht B, Anisetti M, et al. Augmented reality technologies, systems and applications. Multimed Tools Appl 2011;51(1):341–77.
3. Milgram P, Kishino F. A taxonomy of mixed reality visual displays. IEICE Trans Inf Syst 1994;77(12): 1321–9. Available at: https://search.ieice.org/bin/summary.php?id=e77-d_12_1321.
4. Gerrand C. CORR Insights®: can augmented reality be helpful in pelvic bone cancer surgery? an in vitro study. Clin Orthop Relat Res 2018;476(9):1726–7.
5. Sutherland IE. A head-mounted three dimensional display. In: Proceedings of the December 9-11, 1968, Fall Joint Computer Conference, Part I. AFIPS '68 (Fall, part I). New York: Association for Computing Machinery; 1968:757-764. https://doi.org/10.1145/1476589.1476686.
6. Sutherland J, Belec J, Sheikh A, et al. Applying modern virtual and augmented reality technologies to medical images and models. J Digit Imaging 2019;32(1):38–53.

7. Shuhaiber JH. Augmented reality in surgery. Arch Surg 2004;139(2):170–4.

8. Reisman R, Ellis S. Augmented reality for air traffic control towers. In: ACM SIGGRAPH 2003 Sketches & applications. SIGGRAPH '03. San Diego, CA: Association for Computing Machinery; 2003. p. 1. https://doi.org/10.1145/965400.965426.

9. U.S. Air Force photo by Staff Sgt. Samantha Mathison. Fighter Pilot Helmet Display. 2017. Available at: https://www.afrc.af.mil/News/Article-Display/Article/1110726/taking-off-from-the-shoulders-of-giants/. Accessed July 20, 2020.

10. Google "Project Glass" replaces the smartphone with glasses. PCMAG. Available at: https://www.pcmag.com/archive/google-project-glass-replaces-the-smartphone-with-glasses-296284. Accessed July 24, 2020.

11. Gannes L. Next Google Glass tricks include translating the world from your eyes. AllThingsD. Available at: http://allthingsd.com/20131119/new-google-glass-apps-will-translate-the-world-from-your-eyes-and-other-tricks/. Accessed July 24, 2020.

12. HoloLens 2—overview, features, and specs | Microsoft HoloLens. Available at: https://www.microsoft.com/en-us/hololens/hardware. Accessed July 24, 2020.

13. Rankin TM, Slepian MJ, Armstrong DG. Augmented reality in surgery. In: Latifi R, Rhee P, Gruessner RWG, editors. Technological advances in surgery, trauma and critical care. New York: Springer New York; 2015. p. 59–71. https://doi.org/10.1007/978-1-4939-2671-8_6.

14. Kelley TC, Swank ML. Role of navigation in total hip arthroplasty. J Bone Joint Surg Am 2009;91(Suppl 1):153–8.

15. Bae DK, Song SJ. Computer assisted navigation in knee arthroplasty. Clin Orthop Surg 2011;3(4):259–67.

16. Zhou F, Duh HB, Billinghurst M. Trends in augmented reality tracking, interaction and display: a review of ten years of ISMAR. In: September 15 - 18, 2008 7th IEEE/ACM International Symposium on Mixed and Augmented Reality. Cambridge, UK. ieeexplore.ieee.org; 2008. p. 193-202. https://doi.org/10.1109/ISMAR.2008.4637362.

17. Auvinet E, Maillot C, Uzoho C. Augmented reality technology for joint replacement. In: Rivière C, Vendittoli P-A, editors. Personalized hip and knee joint replacement. Cham (Switzerland): Springer International Publishing; 2020. p. 321–8. https://doi.org/10.1007/978-3-030-24243-5_27.

18. Vávra P, Roman J, Zonča P, et al. Recent development of augmented reality in surgery: a review. J Healthc Eng 2017;2017:4574172.

19. Yeniaras E, Navkar NV, Sonmez AE, et al. MR-based real time path planning for cardiac operations with transapical access. Med Image Comput Comput Assist Interv 2011;14(Pt 1): 25–32.

20. Tsutsumi N, Tomikawa M, Uemura M, et al. Image-guided laparoscopic surgery in an open MRI operating theater. Surg Endosc 2013;27(6):2178–84.

21. Sugano N. Computer-assisted orthopaedic surgery and robotic surgery in total hip arthroplasty. Clin Orthop Surg 2013;5(1):1–9.

22. Zheng G, Nolte LP. Computer-assisted orthopedic surgery: current state and future perspective. Front Surg 2015;2:66.

23. Navab N, Heining S-M, Traub J. Camera augmented mobile C-arm (CAMC): calibration, accuracy study, and clinical applications. IEEE Trans Med Imaging 2010;29(7):1412–23.

24. Londei R, Esposito M, Diotte B, et al. Intra-operative augmented reality in distal locking. Int J Comput Assist Radiol Surg 2015;10(9):1395–403.

25. van Duren BH, Sugand K, Wescott R, et al. Augmented reality fluoroscopy simulation of the guide-wire insertion in DHS surgery: A proof of concept study. Med Eng Phys 2018;55:52–9.

26. Hiranaka T, Fujishiro T, Hida Y, et al. Augmented reality: the use of the PicoLinker smart glasses improves wire insertion under fluoroscopy. World J Orthop 2017;8(12):891–4.

27. Befrui N, Fischer M, Fuerst B, et al. 3D augmented reality visualization for navigated osteosynthesis of pelvic fractures. Unfallchirurg 2018;121(4):264–70.

28. Zemirline A, Agnus V, Soler L, et al. Augmented reality-based navigation system for wrist arthroscopy: feasibility. J Wrist Surg 2013;2(4):294–8.

29. Carl B, Bopp M, Saß B, et al. Implementation of augmented reality support in spine surgery. Eur Spine J 2019;28(7):1697–711.

30. Edström E, Burström G, Omar A, et al. Augmented reality surgical navigation in spine surgery to minimize staff radiation exposure. Spine 2020;45(1): E45–53.

31. Elmi-Terander A, Nachabe R, Skulason H, et al. Feasibility and accuracy of thoracolumbar minimally invasive pedicle screw placement with augmented reality navigation technology. Spine 2018;43(14):1018–23.

32. Adams M. Dr. Frank Phillips is first in the world to use augmented reality surgical guidance in minimally invasive spine surgery. OrthoSpineNews. 2020. Available at: https://orthospinenews.com/2020/06/17/dr-frank-phillips-is-first-in-the-world-to-use-augmented-reality-surgical-guidance-in-minimally-invasive-spine-surgery/. Accessed July 24, 2020.

33. National Center for Biotechnology Information. Available at: https://www.ncbi.nlm.nih.gov/. Accessed July 24, 2020.

34. Daines BK, Dennis DA. Gap balancing vs. measured resection technique in total knee arthroplasty. Clin Orthop Surg 2014;6(1):1–8.
35. Mason JB, Fehring TK, Estok R, et al. Meta-analysis of alignment outcomes in computer-assisted total knee arthroplasty surgery. J Arthroplasty 2007;22(8):1097–106.
36. Dennis DA, Channer M, Susman MH, et al. Intramedullary versus extramedullary tibial alignment systems in total knee arthroplasty. J Arthroplasty 1993;8(1):43–7.
37. Tabatabaee RM, Rasouli MR, Maltenfort MG, et al. Computer-assisted total knee arthroplasty: is there a difference between image-based and imageless techniques? J Arthroplasty 2018;33(4):1076–81.
38. Nam D, Weeks KD, Reinhardt KR, et al. Accelerometer-based, portable navigation vs imageless, large-console computer-assisted navigation in total knee arthroplasty: a comparison of radiographic results. J Arthroplasty 2013;28(2):255–61.
39. Pokhrel S, Alsadoon A, Prasad PWC, et al. A novel augmented reality (AR) scheme for knee replacement surgery by considering cutting error accuracy. Int J Med Robot 2019;15(1):e1958.
40. Whitaker H, Halas J. Timing for animation. Boca Raton, FL: CRC Press; 2013. Available at: https://play.google.com/store/books/details?id=yMgqBgAAQBAJ.
41. Wang L, Sun Z, Zhang X, et al. A HoloLens Based Augmented Reality Navigation System for Minimally Invasive Total Knee Arthroplasty. In: Yu H, Liu J, Liu L, et al, editors. Intelligent Robotics and Applications. New York, NY: Springer; 2019. p. 519–30. https://doi.org/10.1007/978-3-030-27529-7_44.
42. Daniel C, Ramos O. Augmented reality for assistance of total knee replacement. J Electr Comput Eng 2016;2016. https://doi.org/10.1155/2016/9358369.
43. Tsukada S, Ogawa H, Nishino M, et al. Augmented reality-based navigation system applied to tibial bone resection in total knee arthroplasty. J Exp Orthop 2019;6(1):44.
44. Parratte S, Price AJ, Jeys LM, et al. Accuracy of a new robotically assisted technique for total knee arthroplasty: a cadaveric study. J Arthroplasty 2019;34(11):2799–803.
45. Pixee Medical develops surgical navigation solutions using an innovative tracking tool. Pixee Medical. Available at: https://www.pixee-medical.com/en/. Accessed July 9, 2020.
46. Pixee Medical : News & events. Pixee Medical. Available at: https://www.pixee-medical.com/en/news-events/. Accessed July 15, 2020.
47. Henry S, Kilian P, Fissette R. Cutting device for the placement of a knee prosthesis. World Patent. 2020. Available at: https://patentimages.storage.googleapis.com/3c/68/fc/6a4da057156618/WO2020099268A1.pdf. Accessed July 15, 2020.
48. VUZIX. Vuzix M400 | Implementing workflow improvements. Available at: https://www.vuzix.com/products/m400-smart-glasses. Accessed July 15, 2020.
49. NextAR. Available at: https://nextar.medacta.com/. Accessed July 15, 2020.
50. Lewinnek GE, Lewis JL, Tarr R, et al. Dislocations after total hip-replacement arthroplasties. J Bone Joint Surg Am 1978;60(2):217–20. Available at: https://www.ncbi.nlm.nih.gov/pubmed/641088.
51. Tezuka T, Heckmann ND, Bodner RJ, et al. Functional safe zone is superior to the Lewinnek safe zone for total hip arthroplasty: why the lewinnek safe zone is not always predictive of stability. J Arthroplasty 2019;34(1):3–8.
52. Fotouhi J, Alexander CP, Unberath M, et al. Plan in 2-D, execute in 3-D: an augmented reality solution for cup placement in total hip arthroplasty. J Med Imaging (Bellingham) 2018;5(2):021205.
53. Sato Y, Sasama T, Sugano N, et al. Intraoperative simulation and planning using a combined acetabular and femoral (CAF) navigation system for total hip replacement. In: Delp SL, DiGoia AM, Jaramaz B, editors. Medical image computing and computer-assisted intervention – MICCAI 2000. Springer Berlin Heidelberg; 2000. p. 1114–25. https://doi.org/10.1007/978-3-540-40899-4_116.
54. Alexander C, Loeb AE, Fotouhi J, et al. Augmented reality for acetabular component placement in direct anterior total hip arthroplasty. J Arthroplasty 2020;35(6):1636–41.e3.
55. Wilson MR, Poolton JM, Malhotra N, et al. Development and validation of a surgical workload measure: the surgery task load index (SURG-TLX). World J Surg 2011;35(9):1961–9.
56. Ogawa H, Hasegawa S, Tsukada S, et al. A pilot study of augmented reality technology applied to the acetabular cup placement during total hip arthroplasty. J Arthroplasty 2018;33(6):1833–7.
57. Ogawa H, Kurosaka K, Sato A, et al. Does an augmented reality-based portable navigation system improve the accuracy of acetabular component orientation during THA? a randomized controlled trial. Clin Orthop Relat Res 2020;478(5):935–43.
58. Murray DW. The definition and measurement of acetabular orientation. J Bone Joint Surg Br 1993;75(2):228–32. Available at: https://www.ncbi.nlm.nih.gov/pubmed/8444942.
59. Kamphuis C, Barsom E, Schijven M, et al. Augmented reality in medical education? Perspect Med Educ 2014;3(4):300–11.
60. Aïm F, Lonjon G, Hannouche D, et al. Effectiveness of virtual reality training in orthopaedic surgery. Arthroscopy 2016;32(1):224–32.

61. Haque S, Srinivasan S. A meta-analysis of the training effectiveness of virtual reality surgical simulators. IEEE Trans Inf Technol Biomed 2006;10(1): 51–8.

62. Ponce BA, Jennings JK, Clay TB, et al. Telementoring: use of augmented reality in orthopaedic education: AAOS exhibit selection. J Bone Joint Surg Am 2014;96(10):e84.

63. Logishetty K, Western L, Morgan R, et al. Can an augmented reality headset improve accuracy of acetabular cup orientation in simulated THA? a randomized trial. Clin Orthop Relat Res 2019;477(5): 1190–9.

64. Condino S, Turini G, Parchi PD, et al. How to build a patient-specific hybrid simulator for orthopaedic open surgery: benefits and limits of mixed-reality using the microsoft holoLens. J Healthc Eng 2018; 2018:5435097.

65. Turini G, Condino S, Parchi PD, et al. A Microsoft HoloLens mixed reality surgical simulator for patient-specific hip arthroplasty training. In: De Paolis LT, Bourdot P, editors. Augmented reality, virtual reality, and computer graphics. New York, NY: Springer; 2018. p. 201–10. https://doi.org/10. 1007/978-3-319-95282-6_15.

66. Kim Y, Kim H, Kim YO. Virtual reality and augmented reality in plastic surgery: a review. Arch Plast Surg 2017;44(3):179–87.

67. Bigart KC, Nahhas CR, Ruzich GP, et al. Does femoral morphology predict the risk of periprosthetic fracture after cementless total hip arthroplasty? J Arthroplasty 2020. https://doi.org/10. 1016/j.arth.2020.02.048.

68. Dugdale M. Wright's Blueprint MR used in shoulder arthroplasty procedure. VRWorldTech. 2020. Available at: https://vrworldtech.com/2020/07/20/wrights-blueprint-mr-used-in-shoulder-arthroplasty-procedure/. Accessed July 21, 2020.

69. Haaker RG, Stockheim M, Kamp M, et al. Computer-assisted navigation increases precision of component placement in total knee arthroplasty. Clin Orthop Relat Res 2005;433:152–9.

70. Kamara E, Berliner ZP, Hepinstall MS, et al. Pin site complications associated with computer-assisted navigation in hip and knee arthroplasty. J Arthroplasty 2017;32(9):2842–6.

71. Matsumoto T, Muratsu H, Kubo S, et al. Intraoperative soft tissue balance reflects minimum 5-year midterm outcomes in cruciate-retaining and posterior-stabilized total knee arthroplasty. J Arthroplasty 2012;27(9):1723–30.

72. Claus D, Fitzgibbon AW. Reliable automatic calibration of a marker-based position tracking system. In: Azada D, editor. 2005 Seventh IEEE Workshops on Applications of Computer Vision (WACV/MOTION'05) - Volume 1. vol. 1. Piscataway, NJ: IEEE publishers; 5-7 January, 2005. Breckenridge, CO: p. 300–5. https://doi.org/10. 1109/ACVMOT.2005.101.

73. Lappin T. C-130 jet: Co-pilot's head-up display panel. 2004. Available at: https://www.flickr.com/photos/49502995517@N01/4136242. Accessed July 24, 2020.

74. Babir N. Apollo 11 astronaut Buzz Aldrin tries out Microsoft HoloLens mixed reality headset 2016. Available at: https://www.flickr.com/photos/nasa-kennedy/29794543715/. Accessed July 24, 2020.

Development and Implementation of International Curricula for Joint Replacement and Preservation

Kokeb Andenmatten[a], Florence Provence[b],
Michael Cunningham, PhD[c], Aresh Sepehri, MD, MSc[d],
Carsten Perka, MD[e], Pipsa Ylänkö[b],
Bassam A. Masri, MD, FRCSC[f],*

KEYWORDS

- Competency-based medical education • Curriculum development • Orthopedics education
- Arthroplasty • Joint preservation

KEY POINTS

- AO Foundation has been delivering education to surgeons worldwide since the early 1960s and adopted a competency-based curriculum approach in 2010.
- The establishment of AO Recon in 2014 was a response to the significant global demand for high-quality arthroplasty education.
- Reports on the implementation of competency-based curricula continue to identify best practices, often from residency programs.

INTRODUCTION

The aging population in many countries is a contributing factor to an ongoing increase in demand for joint arthroplasty.[1] In 2019, 703 million people were at least 65 years old and the United Nations *World Population Aging 2019* report projects the number to double by 2050. The international analysis of total knee arthroplasty (TKA) data from databases and registries in 18 countries by Kurtz and colleagues[2,3] concluded that the demand for TKA significantly increases across the world and also reported young patients may play a role in the future demand for primary and revision surgery. By 2030, in the United States, the numbers of procedures yearly are projected to increase to 572,000 primary total hip arthroplasties and 3.48 million primary TKA.[4] The rise in demand for more arthroplasty procedures and associated complications and periprosthetic fractures leads to rising numbers of surgeons performing these procedures worldwide, and this requires an increase in arthroplasty education.

Arthroplasty Curriculum

In North America, the specific curricular requirements for Orthopedic Surgery Residency and Orthopedic Surgery Fellowships are available on the Accreditation Council for Graduate

[a] AO Foundation - AO Education Institute, Stettbachstrasse 6, Dübendorf 8600, Switzerland; [b] AO Recon, Clavadelerstrasse 8, Davos Platz 7270, Switzerland; [c] AO Foundation - AO Education Institute, Stettbachstrasse 6, Dübendorf 8600, Switzerland; [d] Department of Orthopaedics, University of British Columbia, Diamond Health Care Centre, 11th Floor - 2775 Laurel Street, Vancouver, British Columbia V5Z 1M9, Canada; [e] Charité, University Medicine Berlin, Charitéplatz 1, Berlin 10117, Germany; [f] Department of Orthopaedics, Complex Joint Reconstruction Clinic, Gordon & Leslie Diamond Health Care Centre, University of British Columbia, 3rd Floor, 2775 Laurel Street, Vancouver, British Columbia V5Z 1M9, Canada
* Corresponding author.
E-mail address: bas.masri@ubc.ca

Orthop Clin N Am 52 (2021) 27–39
https://doi.org/10.1016/j.ocl.2020.08.003

Medical Education Web site (www.acgme.org). Program requirements refer to essential educational structures, processes, or resources required across all graduate training programs.[5] Outcome requirements refer to measurable educational outcomes characterized as the knowledge, skills, or attitudes residents or fellows should demonstrate at key points in training. A review of the orthopedic surgery milestones is also available on their Web site. Kellam and colleagues[6] have published Core Competencies for General Orthopedic Surgeons and proposed minimum knowledge and competencies necessary to deliver acute and general orthopedic care as a first step in defining a practice-based standard for training programs and certification groups. Many orthopedic curricula worldwide also contain specific objectives or procedures for arthroplasty (eg, Pakistan, India, Taiwan, Singapore, Indonesia, Greece, Hungary, United Kingdom, EFORT) and some of these describe competencies or milestones for residency programs. The curricula focus on residency requirements leading to board certification, but typically not for post qualification subspecialization or continuing professional development (CPD). The assessment of residents is tied to the qualification process where CPD requirements vary around the world and often require a more general evaluation process rather than a structured assessment tied to set standards and milestones. In some countries, practicing surgeons learn "on the job" from experienced colleagues and from constant exchange with peers. They may also receive education through courses from societies or from industry, and some complete national or international fellowships or observerships. As medical technology and orthopedic techniques continue to evolve throughout a surgeon's career, CPD beyond a surgeon's initial qualifying training is important to ensure patients are provided with the most up-to-date care.

Competency-Based Medical Education

Competency-based medical education (CBME) is an outcomes-based approach to the design, implementation, assessment, and evaluation of medical education programs, using an organized framework of competencies.[7] A competency is an observable ability of a health professional, integrating multiple components such as knowledge, skills, values, and attitudes. Competencies can be assembled like building blocks to facilitate progressive development and they can be measured and assessed. The rationale for CBME is that medical curricula

must ensure that all graduates are competent in all essential domains and that they must be entrusted in delivering the professional activities independently once they have qualified. Competencies provide clear goals for learners and milestones are defined for training programs with the focus on what the learner attains rather than the length of time they are in training. Many CBME concepts are applied to education for qualified surgeons in the form of CPD and continuing medical education (CME). CBME has evolved as a core concept in curriculum development in many specialties over the past 50 years. Competency-based education in orthopedics has been described in several publications in the past decade.[8–11] Nousiainen and colleagues[12] have reported 8-year outcomes following the introduction of CBME in postgraduate medical education at the University of Toronto in Canada.

METHODS

The AO Approach

AO Foundation has been delivering education to surgeons worldwide since the early 1960s and adopted a competency-based curriculum approach in 2010. Through the collaboration of faculty and professional educationalists, this paradigm shift was introduced to its entire educational process from planning through execution to assessment and evaluation. Today, all of its educational events are built around 7 principles of adult education deemed important for postgraduate education and CPD of surgeons.[13] Educational events are designed based on a standardized needs assessment protocol identifying gaps in the knowledge or performance of the participants.[14] The backward planning process is then applied to the educational program development to address the practice and performance gaps of the learners to achieve the best possible outcomes for patients.[15] The delivery of events has shifted from passive teacher-centered setups toward a learner-centered focus with more interactive formats ensuring ample possibilities for feedback and reflection. The AO process for developing a competency-based curriculum for residents was described by Taha[16] in 2015 and has been reported for practicing surgeons in several subspecialty areas.[16–19]

The AO Recon Experience

AO Recon is a global network of orthopedic surgeons delivering best-in-class education in joint replacement and preservation. It was established in 2014 to respond to rising numbers of arthroplasty and periprosthetic fracture cases and the increased need for specialized education and expert advice in this field. AO Recon's goal was to improve the availability of high-quality courses, particularly in countries where practicing surgeons were expanding their practice and have limited availability of effective educational resources. The need for education was supported by responses from more than 4000 surgeons worldwide in an AO Trauma global needs assessment in 2013.[20] AO Recon's global network is surgeon-led with a Steering Board and an Education Forum, which is responsible for AO Recon's education strategy and activities. These groups appoint the surgeon faculty as members of the curriculum taskforces and approve annual event planning. They define the main areas for curriculum development and support the recommendations and implementation of the curricula. The Education Forum decided that competency-based curriculum development was needed to directly impact patient health and meet the diverse and evolving educational needs of joint replacement and preservation surgeons. The Forum decided to start with hip and knee and to expand into the other areas over several years. In this article, we share best practices and experiences from the development of their 4 curricula in joint replacement and reconstruction.

AO Recon Curriculum Development Process

A taskforce of 3 or more expert surgeons was appointed and an educationalist from the AO Education Institute supported a structured process for developing each competency-based curriculum through a series of face-to-face and online meetings. The goal of each taskforce was to design and deliver a range of educational events for each target audience that would enable successful learning with measurable outcomes. This methodology is based on a standardized multi-step approach in medical education with 3 main phases: (1) curriculum design, (2) content development, and (3) continuous improvement.

To build education that directly impacts patient health, we follow a backward planning process as the first step in curriculum development. We identify the patient problems that reconstructive surgeons address and identify the current performance gaps. We define the competencies (abilities) that surgeons must have to address and avoid these problems. Based on these competencies and specific learning objectives, we design educational activities to directly impact corresponding clinical

performance and so improve patient health in the relevant areas. Our process follows 12 steps in 3 phases as described in the following text.

Design Phase

Step 1 – Identify the patient problems.

We asked the experts to describe the most common and most critical patient and clinical problems based on their experience and published data and references. The emphasis is placed on the patient during all phases of care and this process also defines the scope of the curriculum.

- Output: Prioritized lists of patient problems related to presentation, treatment, and postoperative care.
- Examples from hip and knee curriculum:
  - Pain, loss of function, limping, and complications due to degenerative conditions and trauma
- Examples from shoulder arthroplasty curriculum:
  - Pain, weakness, limited motion, and instability related to degenerative conditions and trauma

Step 2 – Identify the target audiences to be addressed.

We first described the surgeons who are responsible for managing the patient and their specific patient or clinical problems. These are our target audiences, and each group has specific needs and characteristics based on their level of experience and their practice setting.

- Output: Descriptions and characteristics of the main target audience groups.
- Examples from hip and knee arthroplasty (principles level): Newly certified orthopedic surgeons and advanced orthopedic surgical trainees.
- Examples from periprosthetic fractures (complex level): Senior, experienced (more than 5 years) consultant/practicing surgeons (general orthopedic surgeons, fracture specialists, arthroplasty specialists, surgeons experienced with both trauma and arthroplasty).

Step 3 – Identify the performance gaps.

We did this by identifying the gaps in care that may exist in regard to managing the patient problems and then describing what the surgeon must do to optimize patient outcomes.

- Output: Descriptions of what the surgeons must do to provide optimal

patient care (to address any identified gaps).
- Examples from hip joint preservation:
  - Identify the basic pathology and the cause of why a hip is wearing out
  - Describe the advanced radiologic modality options and when and how they can help
- Examples from shoulder arthroplasty:
  - Assess the patient lifestyle, occupational needs, social situation, comorbidities, and so forth, and outcome expectations to decide the treatment options
  - Follow-up the patient to continually reassess the outcomes and adjust the plan when necessary

Step 4 – Define competencies as a framework for all education.

Based on the statements of what the surgeon must do to avoid the performance gaps, we define the competencies that will be the framework for all our education.

- Output: Competencies that we will build all educational offerings around. In our curricula, the number of competencies usually ranges from 6 to 12 depending on the topic area.
- Examples from hip and knee (principles level):
  - Competency 4. Anticipate, recognize, and stratify potential complications.
  - Competency 5. Describe and discuss safe and effective procedures for primary arthroplasty.
- Examples from shoulder arthroplasty:
  - Competency 1. Assess the symptoms for the presenting pathologies using clinical history, examination, and imaging studies.
  - Competency 8. Follow up with the patient to continually reassess the outcomes and adjust the plan when necessary.

Step 5 – Deconstruct the competencies to identify learning objectives.

Each competency was deconstructed into a unique set of knowledge, skill, and attitude components that are our learning objectives. This deconstruction enables us to group objectives and select the most appropriate educational method to achieve these.

- Output: Knowledge, skill, and attitude components for each competency.

- Examples knee joint preservation:
  - Plan a knee osteotomy (skill)
  - Describe when and how to perform an anterior cruciate ligament reconstruction (knowledge)
- Examples from complex hip and knee:
  - Perform intraoperative checks (trialing) and ensure that it reflects the preoperative plan (skill)
  - Recognize that if the patient says there is a problem, there IS a problem to be addressed (attitude)

Step 6 – Identify the procedures that should be addressed.

We identified the operative and nonoperative procedures that our target audiences should know or perform, with the steps and associated complications, and to identify those that should be referred to another expert. We then decided how we could address each procedure in our education based on Miller's levels of outcomes and assessment (knows, knows how, shows how, does).[21]

- Output: A categorized description of operative and nonoperative procedures to be addressed in simulations and other educational activities for each specific target audience.
- Examples from hip and knee (complex level): revision hip procedures, revision knee, complications management.
- Examples from shoulder arthroplasty (principles level): total shoulder arthroplasty (with or without glenoid deformity), primary reverse shoulder arthroplasty.

Development Phase
Step 7 – Select delivery methods.

The group first selected and grouped the learning objectives that would be addressed and based on the level of outcome an appropriate corresponding delivery method was chosen. We use a combination of lecture presentations (including case based and plenary variants), small group discussions, and simulations (eg, practical exercises, anatomic laboratory procedures), and other educational methods to deliver our courses and other events (Fig. 1).

- Output: A plan of activities to address the curriculum competencies with specific learning objectives, defined take-home messages, and a recommended time allocation.

Step 8 – Develop event programs.

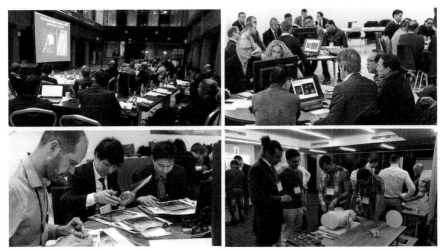

Fig. 1. Main educational methods used in our face-to-face courses: presentations and plenary discussions, small group discussions, meet the experts (example shows planning), and simulations (eg, skills stations, practical exercises).

Based on the taskforce's selection of activities to deliver the learning objectives, educational events are then defined (eg, courses, seminars, webinars). Our programs are designed to align with local CME requirements and best practices in CPD.

- Output: A standardized program showing the sequenced and timed educational activities with defined learning objectives, structured into modules and days with defined supporting materials.
- Examples from periprosthetic fractures: a 2-day course with lectures, small group case discussions, and dry bone practical exercises (2.5-day course when an anatomic specimen laboratory to replace the dry bone practical exercises).
- Examples from hip and knee joint preservation: 1 day of presentations, small group discussions, and practical exercises to integrate in complex hip and complex knee course.

Step 9 – Prepare faculty support material and resources.

We developed a full supporting package for all faculty to deliver their assigned educational activity and for the chairperson and organizer to plan and run the overall event. This includes case libraries, learning objectives and outlines, some standardized lectures, guides for hands-on activities (skills laboratory, dry bone or anatomic specimen laboratory exercises), and assessment and evaluation tools.

- Output: A full and dedicated faculty support package.

- Examples from hip and knee (principles level): Videos and posters of all skills stations and a booklet for participants.
- Examples from periprosthetic fractures: A set of multiple-choice assessment questions to implement before each course to gather information on the needs of the participants who will attend.

Step 10 – Conduct and analyze pre-event assessment and post-event evaluation.

Pre-event assessment

Our pre-course assessment is conducted several days before each event to provide information about the educational needs (gaps scores) and practice profile of the participants (years of experience, caseload, hospital setting).[22] This helps the faculty to finetune the content to the specific audience at each event. For every type of AO Recon course, participants have consistently shown good motivation to learn (gap scores between 1 and 2.5 between their self-assessed present and desired levels of ability) (example shown in **Fig. 2**). This confirms the educational need for all competencies in the planned target audiences. Data from all individual courses are summarized to detect trends and regional differences and to help our committees to plan future events and locations (example shown in **Fig. 3**).

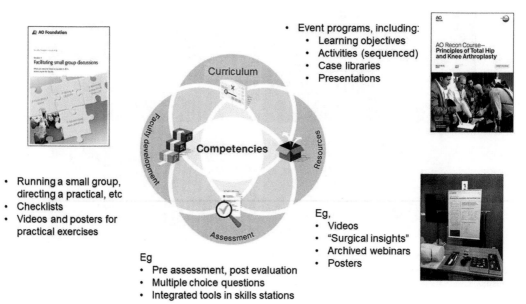

Fig. 2. Our competency-based approach to quality education (4 main components).

Post-event evaluation

On the last day of the course, participants complete a set of evaluation questions to rate the impact of the course, the content, the faculty, the level of commercial bias, and the usefulness of the specific activities (lectures, discussion groups, and practical exercises). Key information is reported to the chairpersons for each individual event.[22] Data from all events are combined per curriculum to help taskforces and regions to identify any changes that need to be made to, for example, the curriculum or implementation (examples shown in **Fig. 4, Table 1**).

Maintenance and Improvement Phase
Step 11 – Review all evaluation and assessment data and feedback.

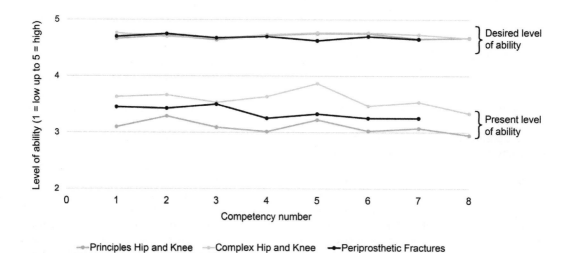

Fig. 3. Motivation to learn for various courses over multiple years (average gap scores between participant self-assessed present and desired levels of ability).

The chairperson and faculty analyze the data from every individual event. In addition, each curriculum taskforce reviews data from new initiatives and conducts a yearly review of all related data. This identifies areas to update in terms of content and faculty support material based on evaluation and assessment of data and feedback regarding what went well and what we could do differently.

- Output: Decisions for new content or events.
- Examples from hip and knee (principles level): Analysis of feedback from first 2 years of the principles course covering primary and revision hip and knee procedures resulting in some changes to the curriculum.
- Examples from hip and knee (complex level): Analysis of feedback requesting the integration of "hands-on" components.

Step 12 – Update the curriculum and events when required or to meet new needs.

Based on data analysis and new needs, each taskforce updates their competency-based curriculum each year and defines and changes or additions to the educational events. Feedback from all regions is considered and current literature and new developments are analyzed in the process.

- Output: Updated curriculum or events.

- Examples from hip and knee (principles level): Addition of the AO Recon skills laboratory to integrate hands-on skills training after the first 2 years of the course.
- Examples from hip and knee (complex level): Addition of hands-on dry bone practical exercises and anatomy laboratory components after 1 year of the new complex course, and create 2 courses, 1 specific for the hip and 1 for the knee that integrate joint preservation into each of the 2 new courses.

RESULTS
Curriculum Output and Milestones
Over 5 years, 4 taskforces in AO Recon have developed new competency-based curricula for hip and knee arthroplasty, periprosthetic fractures, shoulder arthroplasty, and joint preservation (Fig. 5). A series of specific 1.5-day to 2.5-day face-to-face courses have been designed to meet defined competencies and learning objectives using a combination of presentations, small group discussions, dry bone practical exercises or anatomic laboratory procedures, and other educational methods. Our courses are designed for 24 to 64 participants and are usually supported by 2 chairpersons and 8 to 12 faculty members (some local and some international). All events have a registration process and a cost-recovery fee and are open to surgeons worldwide. Evaluation data

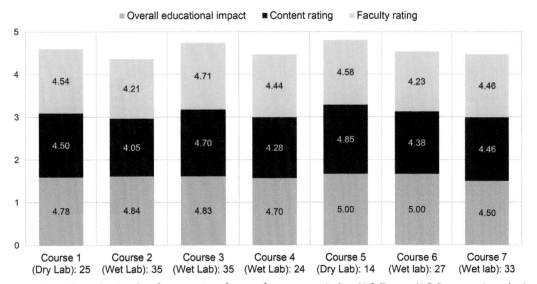

Fig. 4. Example evaluation data from a series of events from one curriculum (AO Trauma/AO Recon periprosthetic fractures of the hip and knee) over 3 years in Europe, Middle East, and Latin America.

Table 1
Self-assessed levels of participant expertise on hip and knee procedures showing differences in Principles and Complex courses in our educational regions (helps identify regions and countries where Complex hip or knee only courses may be more appropriate than the combined course)

Courses by region	Hip Replacement, %				Knee Replacement, %			
	None	Low	Medium	High	None	Low	Medium	High
Principles								
Asia Pacific (8 courses)	11	42	42	6	11	39	41	9
Latin America (6 courses)	3	34	50	13	16	36	37	11
Europe and Southern Africa (5 courses)	8	42	43	8	9	49	35	8
Middle East and Northern Africa (3 courses)	4	41	50	5	6	26	55	13
Complex								
Asia Pacific (2 courses)	2	8	46	35	2	16	60	24
Latin America (1 course)	7	52	33	7	22	33	30	15
Europe and Southern Africa (1 course)	5	16	42	37	5	11	53	32
Middle East and Northern Africa (1 course)	0	19	63	19	0	12	52	36
Global (3 courses)	0	8	56	36	2	11	46	41

have been gathered and analyzed as a standard component of implementation. The structured planning and design of educational events has resulted in principles-focused education that meets the needs of surgeons in many regions of the world. Educational content has recently been integrated on topics such as infection and joint preservation and will continue to evolve to incorporate other high demand topics and novel surgical techniques. Future topics include soft tissue management, electronic planning, and navigation-assisted surgery.

Themes arising from feedback
At every course, feedback and suggestions are gathered from participants, faculty, and task-force members. Hundreds of comments are analyzed every year for each curriculum to identify recurring themes to help guide future planning. Example statements and suggestions for further development included:

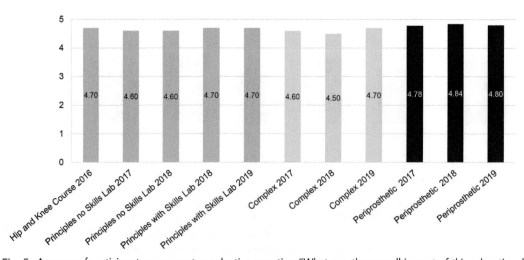

Fig. 5. Average of participant responses to evaluation question "What was the overall impact of this educational event?" (scale of 1–5, where 1 = "I did not learn anything new " up to 5 = "I learned something new and plan to use it in my practice", by course type over 4 years).

Participants

- A highly valuable course, directly from the experts in the field. It starts with basic and ends with the controversies in arthroplasty.
- Interesting case discussions and very good that you see different opinions on arthroplasty details, so that you can make up your one choice.
- The 2-day course first got me interested because of the mixture of evidence-based lectures and case discussions in small groups. And the practical part at the skill stations turned out to be the most effective new aspect in learning arthroplasty surgery.

Faculty

- The demand for arthroplasty will continue to increase globally, education and research will be critical to improve the delivery of care to the patients. Patients' expectations will continue to go up and physicians must be prepared to meet those demands.
- Smaller size courses allow learners to be more actively involved in small groups.
- Split the exercises and have more step by step; we could pair surgeons with trauma and arthroplasty expertise in laboratories in the periprosthetic course.
- The courses enable participants to share their regional realities, which makes the courses more interesting to hear from local and international faculty in order to further standardize education.
- "Local cases would be better" although some other faculty reported "I can use any well documented educational case to focus on the principles and key messages."

Taskforce members

- Faculty need to agree on the key messages and ways to teach in advance (videos are a great way to standardize messages and a master demo can follow the same steps).
- When we add skills and practical procedures, we must make sure that the indications and decision making for all the procedures are not reduced from the curriculum.
- We could provide more regionally focused content to better meet local needs (we can expand our case library with regional topics over time).
- The moderator should ensure the take-home messages are delivered after plenary discussions.

Lessons learned

The establishment of AO Recon in 2014 was a response to the significant global demand for high-quality arthroplasty education. The evolution of our educational initiatives and curricula are summarized in Table 2. Each development in the curriculum required decision making from an international panel of surgeon experts supported by educationalists and managers to plan implementation. Curriculum taskforces have been established since the early years and to design the first course in 2015. The first offering has evolved into a range of courses with hands-on components and now covers principles and complex levels and a wide range of subspecialty offerings. Due to the global lockdown in 2020, AO Recon adapted quickly to expand its digital offerings based on the curricula in English, Chinese, and Spanish. Looking forward, we plan to build more engaging online courses and to explore blended learning combining online and face-to-face components. Below, we share examples of some the most interesting questions that taskforces encountered during the evolution of the initiative and how the taskforces made their decisions and plans.

What Amount of Standardization Is Optimal?
Although most of our programs are very standardized, flexibility is needed to offer the local event chairperson and faculty to cater the course to the local needs of the participants.

When Should Hands-on Skills Components Be Added?
It is difficult to teach "shows how" competencies using didactic tools. This led to the evolution of the course programs with the development and addition of skills stations and practical exercises and anatomy laboratories in many of the courses and is reported in a separate article in this journal.[23]

What Do We Need to Do to Prepare and Support the Faculty?
With a competency-based curriculum, educational methods may be selected where some faculty members have less experience than others (eg, moderating a small group discussion, conducting a skill station with 6 or 8 successive groups of participants, providing feedback in a

Table 2
Evolution of AO Recon educational initiatives and curricula over 5 years

Education and Specific Curriculum	2015	2016	2017	2018	2019	2020[a]
Overall						
Symposia at congresses	6	11	8	9	7	10
Seminars and courses	3	6	13	13	22	36
Online events			1	3	3	4
Hip and knee arthroplasty						
Curriculum taskforce	2 members	2 members	3 members	3 members	3 members	9 members
Principles courses (without Skills Laboratory)	3	6	11	5	2	
Principles courses (with Skills Laboratory)				3	9	19
Complex courses (without exercises)			1	1		
Complex courses (with dry bone or preoperative planning practical exercises)				2	5	7
Complex courses (with anatomy laboratory)					1	3
Complex hip courses – arthroplasty and joint preservation						4 members Planning phase
Complex knee courses – arthroplasty and joint preservation						2 members Planning phase
Periprosthetic fractures (in cooperation with AO Trauma, events listed here organized by AO Recon)						
Curriculum taskforce		4 members	4 members	4 members	4 members	4 members
Courses (with dry bone practical exercises)			1		1	
Courses (with anatomy laboratory)				1	1	2
Shoulder arthroplasty						
Curriculum taskforce			2 members	2 members	4 members	4 members
Symposia		1		2	2	2
Principles seminars					1	1
Principles course						2
Online						
Webinars			1	2	2	4
Other						
Global needs assessment					Done	
AO Recon fellowships						Planned
Surgical Insights article series	1	1	1	1	2	3

[a] Based on original event planning approved in 2019. The numbers have been constantly changing due to the impact of COVID-19. This has not been reflected in the above numbers.

structured and objective manner). Faculty support with educational resources is crucial to ensure smooth delivery of such a curriculum. Related to the addition of practical exercises, all faculty must review the teaching videos and content in advance of each event and agree to those core procedures and messages.

Needs assessment

We conducted an online needs assessment in 2019 and 413 surgeons responded from 80 countries. We asked surgeons to "rate your need for further education in each of the areas below over the next 2 to 3 years." Seventy percent reported a "medium" or "high" level of need for education on primary hip arthroplasty, 80% for revision procedures. The percentages for primary and revision knee were 61% and 66% the percentages for shoulder arthroplasty were 55% and 48%. Joint preservation, infection, soft tissue, and periprosthetic were reported as a medium or high need by the majority. These findings suggest that there is an ongoing need for education on primary and revision arthroplasty and related areas in many countries for both residents and qualified surgeons.

DISCUSSION

A recent review reconfirms the growth in the numbers of procedures worldwide and identifies broad variation in utilization trends of hip and knee arthroplasty in different countries related to economic and social differences.[23] The investigators suggest that comparing national registers is crucial to determine variations in practices and to identify prospective topics for future analysis and therefore also education. Two recent reports also shows the challenges of implementing an arthroplasty program in a developing country.[24,25] The patient demographics and lack of resources in some countries mean that arthroplasty procedures are more challenging and have a higher chance of revision surgery or complications. Education must address those topics adequately by integrating them into entry level primary prosthesis training.

Reports on the implementation of competency-based curricula continue to identify best practices, often from residency programs. Wagner and colleagues[26] report the main challenges as a need for new assessment tools that assess competency and provide the learner with formative feedback and difficulty with implementation due to a lack of faculty or administrative support, and a lack of knowledge on how to transition to CBME. Fraser and colleagues[26] suggest faculty development activities must continue until all faculty demonstrate an acceptable level of competence (and faculty buy-in is paramount to the successful delivery of any program that is not mandatory). Karthikeyan and Pulimoottil[27] highlights the important role that intra-departmental and inter-institutional cross-communication and exchange of ideas in workshops and personal communication play in reaching consensus and finding relevant solutions to common problems.[28] Harris and colleagues recently shared experiences from the introduction of competency-based models, which has progressed from a single orthopedic surgery training program at the University of Toronto through implementation across all 68 disciplines overseen by the Royal College of Physicians and Surgeons of Canada. Sergeant and colleagues[29] summarize that competency-based CPD is "envisioned to place health needs and patient outcomes at the center of a system that will be guided by a set of competencies to enhance the quality of practice and the safety of the health system." They propose that the "future CPD system should be: grounded in the everyday workplace, integrated into the health care system, oriented to patient outcomes, guided by multiple sources of performance and outcome data, and team-based, and should use the principles and strategies of quality improvement (QI)". Opportunities for international collaboration and education will continue in the areas of arthroplasty and joint preservation and best practices should be shared.

CLINICS CARE POINTS

- Competency-based medical education (CBME) is a core concept in curriculum development in many specialties.
- A contributing factor to an ongoing increase in demand for joint arthroplasty is the aging population in many countries.
- Young patients may play a role in the future demand for primary and revision surgery.
- There is broad variation in the trends in hip and knee arthroplasty and complications/revisions in different countries related to economic and resource differences.
- Exchanging ideas and reaching consensus helps find relevant solutions to common problems.

ACKNOWLEDGMENTS

Acknowledgments and funding for AO Recon curriculum development

Thanks to all the surgeon faculty in the curriculum taskforces below and to all the faculty who have supported them in development and implementation and all the participants who have provided feedback:

- Hip and knee arthroplasty: Michael Huo (US), Robert Hube (Germany), Bassam Masri (Canada), Carsten Perka (Germany, 2014–2016), Fares Haddad (UK, 2014–2016)
- Periprosthetic fractures: Karl Stoffel (Switzerland), Luigi Zagra (Italy), Mark Reilly (US), Gijs van Hellemondt (Netherlands), Vincenzo Giordano (Brazil)
- Shoulder arthroplasty: Paul Favorito (US), Chunyan Jiang (China), Stefaan Nijs (Belgium), Markus Scheibel (Switzerland)
- Joint preservation: Sam Oussedik (UK), Matthieu Ollivier (France), Moritz Tannast (Switzerland), Michael Dienst (Germany), Paul Beaule (Canada), George Grammatopoulos (Canada)

Thanks also to AO Recon and the AO Education Institute. Thanks to DePuy Synthes for an educational grant that provided funding for the development and for their support in implementing hands-on practical exercises.

DISCLOSURE

The authors have no conflicts of interest to disclose.

REFERENCES

1. United Nations, Department of Economic and Social Affairs, Population Division. World population ageing 2019 2020. ST/ESA/SER.A/444. Available at: https://www.un.org/en/development/desa/population/publications/pdf/ageing/WorldPopulationAgeing2019-Highlights.pdf.
2. Kurtz SM, Ong KL, Lau E, et al. International survey of primary and revision total knee replacement. Int Orthop 2011;35(12):1783–9.
3. Kurtz SM, Lau E, Ong K, et al. Future young patient demand for primary and revision joint replacement: national projections from 2010 to 2030. Clin Orthop Relat Res 2009;467(10):2606–12.
4. Kurtz SM, Ong K, Lau E, et al. Projections of primary and revision hip and knee arthroplasty in the United States from 2005 to 2030. J Bone Joint Surg Am 2007;89(4):780–5.
5. Potts JR 3rd. Assessment of Competence: The Accreditation Council for Graduate Medical Education/Residency Review Committee Perspective. Surg Clin North Am 2016;96(1):15–24.
6. Kellam JF, Archibald D, Barber J, et al. on behalf of the General Orthopaedic Competency Task Force. The Core Competencies for General Orthopaedic Surgeons. The J Bone Joint Surg 2017;99(2):175–81.
7. Frank JR, Snell LS, ten Cate O, et al. Competency-based medical education: theory to practice. Med Teach 2010;32:638–45.
8. Alman BA, Ferguson P, Kraemer W, et al. Competency-based education: a new model for teaching orthopaedics. Instr Course Lect 2013;62:565–9.
9. Ferguson P, Kraemer W, Nousiainen M, et al. Three-year experience with an innovative, modular competency-based curriculum for orthopaedic training. J Bone Joint Surg Am 2013;95:1661–6.
10. Dietl CA, Russell JC. Effect of process changes in surgical training on quantitative outcomes from surgery residency programs. J Surg Educ 2016; 73(5):807–18.
11. Joyce BL, McHale K. Curriculum Design for Competency-Based Education in Orthopaedics. In: Dougherty P, Joyce B, editors. The Orthopedic Educator. Springer: Cham; 2018. https://doi.org/10.1007/978-3-319-62944-5_3.
12. Nousiainen MT, Mironova P, Hynes M, et al. 8-year outcomes of a competency-based residency training program in orthopaedic surgery. Med Teach 2018;18:1–13.
13. Rüetschi U, Baumgaertner M, Kapatkin A, et al. The journey to competency-based education. (Under review). 2021.
14. Fox R, Miner C. Motivation and the facilitation of change, learning and participation in educational programs for health professionals. J Cont Educ Health Prof 1999;19:132–41.
15. Moore DE Jr, Green JS, Gallis HA. Achieving desired results and improved outcomes: integrating planning and assessment throughout learning activities. J Contin Educ Health Prof 2009;29:1–15.
16. Taha W. A guide to developing a competency-based curriculum for a residency training program - an Orthopaedic prospective. J Taibah Univ Med Sci 2015;10(1):109–15. https://doi.org/10.1016/j.jtumed.2015.02.004.
17. Shaye DA, Tollefson T, Shah I, et al. Backward planning a craniomaxillofacial trauma curriculum for the surgical workforce in low-resource settings. World J Surg 2018;42(11):3514–9.
18. Calero-Martinez SA, Matula C, Peraud A, et al. Development and assessment of competency-based neurotrauma course curriculum for international neurosurgery residents and neurosurgeons. Neurosurg Focus 2020;48(3):E13.
19. Schmidt FA, Wong T, Kirnaz S, et al. Development of a curriculum for minimally invasive spine surgery (MISS). Glob Spine J 2020;10(2 Suppl): 122S–5S.
20. Buckley R, Brink P, Kojima K, et al. International needs analysis in orthopaedic trauma for practising

surgeons with a 3-year review of resulting actions. J Eur CME 2017;6(1):1398555.

21. Miller GE. The assessment of clinical skills/competence/performance. Acad Med J Assoc Am Med Colleges 1990;65(9 Suppl):S63–7.

22. Ghidinelli M, Cunningham M, Uhlmann M, et al. Designing and implementing a harmonized evaluation and assessment system for educational events worldwide (in publication 2021).

23. Sepehri A, von Roth P, Stoffel K, et al. Surgical skills training using simulation for basic and complex hip and knee arthroplasty (in publication 2021).

24. Abdelaal MS, Restrepo C, Sharkey PF. Global perspectives on arthroplasty of hip and knee joints. Orthop Clin North Am 2020;51(2):169–76.

25. Pedneault C, St George S, Masri BA. Challenges to implementing total joint replacement programs in developing countries. Orthop Clin North Am 2020;51(2):131–9.

26. Wagner N, Fahim C, Dunn K, et al. Otolaryngology residency education: a scoping review on the shift towards competency-based medical education. Clin Otolaryngol 2017;42(3):564–72.

27. Fraser AB, Stodel EJ, Jee R, et al. Preparing anesthesiology faculty for competency-based medical education. Introduction de la formation médicale fondée sur les compétences en anesthésiologie: comment préparer le corps professoral? Can J Anaesth 2016;63(12):1364–73.

28. Karthikeyan P, Pulimoottil DT. Design and implementation of competency based postgraduate medical education in otorhinolaryngology: the pilot experience in India. Indian J Otolaryngol Head Neck Surg 2019;71(Suppl 1):671–8.

29. Harris KA, Nousiainen MT, Reznick R. Competency-based resident education-the Canadian perspective. Surgery 2020;167(4):681–4.

Physician Wellness in Orthopedic Surgery
Challenges and Solutions

Jeffrey M. Smith, MD, CPC[a],*, Eric A. Boe, DO, MS[b],
Ryan Will, MD[c]

KEYWORDS

- Wellness • Well-being • Ergonomics • Burnout • Emotional exhaustion • Moral injury
- Orthopedic surgery

KEY POINTS

- The growing epidemic of physician burnout, the rate of which is 34% within orthopedic surgery, suggests that a change is needed.
- Our aim is to define four main components of wellness (physical, mental, emotional, and spiritual) and offer potential wellness habits readers can apply to their own lives.
- If you want to experience wellness, you need to practice wellness habits.

INTRODUCTION

A career in orthopedic surgery attracts the best and brightest medical students. Physicians are passion-driven professionals, hard-wired to respond to intrinsic motivators, such as helping patients, rather than extrinsic incentives, such as financial success.[1] In medical school and residency, they learn how to care for patients and sacrifice the equally important task of learning to care for themselves. The growing epidemic of physician burnout, the rate of which is 34% within orthopedic surgery, suggests that a change is needed.[2] Resilience, wellness, or well-being are the factors that determine career satisfaction and longevity. Rather than looking at surgeon wellness as a matter of self-preservation, one needs to focus on surgeon wellness as a mechanism to thrive in such a demanding career. Orthopedic surgeons have been modeled and taught maladaptive habits and behaviors during training. These negative habits prepare surgeons poorly for future practice. The key is to unlearn negative habits and learn new positive habits.

By the time education and residency are completed, an orthopedic surgeon is usually in their late 20s or early 30s. Once training is complete, new stresses await. Many new surgeons have substantial debt, minimal business awareness, and often experience disruptions in family and social connections brought on by geographic relocation. After becoming an attending surgeon, new challenges can include autonomy issues, work-life balance problems, and increased medicolegal concerns. Ideal personality qualities that make successful surgeons can lead to overwork and work-life balance issues, ultimately increasing risk for physician burnout.[3]

We want to help put an end to this vicious cycle. In this article, we advance four main components of physician wellness (physical, mental, emotional, and spiritual) and offer simple steps all orthopedic surgeons can take to address their well-being.

THE FOUR COMPONENTS OF WELLNESS

Wellness is defined as the quality or state of being in good health, especially as an actively

[a] Orthopaedic Trauma & Fracture Specialists Medical Corp., 3750 Convoy Street, Suite #201, San Diego, CA 92111, USA; [b] Unite Orthopaedics Foundation, 3750 Convoy Street, Suite 201, San Diego, CA 92111, USA; [c] Olympia Orthopedic Associates, 615 Lilly Road, Suite #120, Olympia, WA 98506, USA
* Corresponding author.
E-mail address: jeff@surgeonmasters.com

Orthop Clin N Am 52 (2021) 41–52
https://doi.org/10.1016/j.ocl.2020.08.004
0030-5898/21/© 2020 Elsevier Inc. All rights reserved.

sought goal. Wellness is also related to prevention and recovery from acute and chronic injuries. Our aim is to define four main components of wellness (physical, mental, emotional, and spiritual) and offer potential solutions readers can apply to their own lives. It is important to understand that the measure of well-being in any of these areas can be enhanced, diminished, or maintained over time. A surgeon's state of wellness can also ebb and flow based on current events or circumstances in their life. All of these wellness components overlap and interconnect. Understanding the connectedness of each component can help lay a strong foundation on which to grow. From that strong base, one is better able to manage the inevitable highs and lows of a long career in orthopedic surgery.

PHYSICAL WELLNESS

When we talk about wellness, physical wellness is often the first that comes to mind for many physicians and surgeons. This area of wellness encompasses nutrition, exercise, and other self-care, and the prevention or management of acute and chronic physical injuries. This is the base of the pyramid on which the other wellness domains are built. There are many simple preventative measures we can all take to improve our physical wellness. Although we have significant knowledge in these areas, many have difficulty applying this knowledge to their own lives. Self-sacrifice and the principle that the "patient always comes first" are strongly pronounced in the culture of surgery. When one is mentally and physically drained at the end of a long day, finding the energy to incorporate the following recommendations may seem taxing. Our hope is that orthopedic surgery will appreciate the science behind physical optimal performance, similar to the preparation that professional athletes use. We hope that orthopedic surgeons will implement the principle of putting our own oxygen mask on first and see the personal benefits of including these as considerations for physical wellness (Table 1).

Exercise

Many orthopedic surgeons come from a background of athletics or physical activity. Various factors lead to the progressive decline in exercise: normal aging, physical injury, the distractions of starting and raising a family, or simply lack of time and energy. Although orthopedic surgeons fully understand the benefit of exercise

for their patients, perhaps we should be writing ourselves a home exercise program for our own physical preservation. Current Centers for Disease Control and Prevention (CDC) guidelines for adults recommend at least 150 minutes of moderate-intensity aerobic physical activity, or 75 minutes of vigorous-intensity physical activity, or an equivalent combination each week. The guidelines also recommend that adults be active for at least 60 minutes each day.[4]

It is worthwhile to highlight that the benefits of physical exercise go beyond physical

Table 1 Physical wellness challenges and solutions	
Challenges	**Solutions**
Eating habits	Reduce sodium, fat
	Balanced diet
	Increase healthy options, decrease unhealthy options
	Hydration: 2.7 L/d for women, 3.7 L/d for men
	When hungry, drink water
Physical activity	>150 min of moderate-intensity or 75 min of vigorous-intensity aerobic exercises/wk
	Active additionally for 1 h daily
	Strengthening, stretching, and balance exercises
	Cross-training
Sleep	Ideally, 7–9 h of sleep
	As much sleep as possible if <7 h
	Power naps 15–30 min
	Presleep (9 h each night before taking call)
	Timing of caffeine, alcohol, and nicotine before sleep matters
	Minimize blue light before sleep
Acute/ chronic musculo-skeletal injuries	Optimum patient table height (operating room table height to maintain most instrument handles with arm and elbow angle 90°–120°)
	Surgeon posture: neck flexion ≤25°, lumber spine neutral flexion
	Antifatigue mats
	Intraoperative targeted stretch microbreaks

wellness. For example, brain-derived neurotrophic factor is an important molecule and plays a dominant role in mediating the beneficial cognitive effects of physical activity.[5] Aerobic exercise leads to release of brain-derived neurotrophic factor from the brain increasing angiogenesis and hippocampal volume by up to 12%.[6,7] Studies have also shown other benefits with increased brain-derived neurotrophic factor levels including decreased morbidity and mortality; protection against the normal cognitive decline of aging and reduction of the incidence of Alzheimer disease by 30% to 40%[8]; and improved memory, motor skills, and executable functions.[9] An acute exercise session also decreases stress, improves cognitive functions and processing, and improves mood state for up to 24 hours.[10] A recent study showed that only 55% of orthopedic surgeons participated in exercise recommended by CDC guidelines. However, this group of surgeons that followed CDC guidelines for activity had significantly increased overall quality of life scores, physical quality of life scores, and lower burnout rate compared with surgeons who did not follow CDC guidelines for physical activity.[5]

Physical exercise for orthopedic surgeons should account for existing medical conditions. It should include aerobic conditioning, and strengthening, flexibility, and balance. There are significant benefits to cross-training for the prevention of overuse injuries, and for addressing a broader set of musculoskeletal tissues. Physical exercise evolves through the life of an orthopedic surgeon in residency, early, middle, and late career. Physical exercise can come in many forms, and it does not have to be of the same duration nor in the same intensity as medical or nonmedical colleagues, family members, or celebrities. It could be as simple as stretching, going for a walk around the block, or a couple of push-ups. The most important part is to commit to some form of exercise on a routine basis.

Sleep

Sleep deprivation is part of the historical culture in orthopedic surgery training and even many orthopedic careers. Surgeons do not have to resign themselves to the negative consequences of sleep deprivation. Although controversy exists over the ideal amount of nightly sleep or rest, a consensus study points to all adults getting a minimum amount of 7 hours, which is hard to come by in high-stress occupations, such as orthopedic surgery.[11] The most

important consideration of sleep is to sleep long enough to get adequate rapid eye movement sleep.[11]

Many surgeons have difficulty getting a sufficient amount of sleep each night because of long workdays, case preparation, other leadership responsibilities, postcase or precase anxiety, practice-related or on-call nighttime telephone calls, and much more. Some even have sleep impairment because of mental health issues, such as depression, secondary traumatic stress, anxiety, or because of personal family demands. Some surgeons get so good at limiting sleep during training and early career that they continue to purposely get limited sleep. Unfortunately, insufficient sleep syndrome, defined as voluntarily getting less than 7 hours of sleep each night, has significant changes in morbidity and mortality.[12] Insufficient sleep syndrome sufferers have a 12% increase in all-cause mortality, and several studies show increased risk of hypertension, obesity, metabolic syndrome, and overall increase in the risk of cardiovascular morbidity and mortality.[13,14] For most surgeons, including some who think that they tolerate it, sleep deprivation is also strongly associated with cognitive abnormalities: neurobehavioral deficits including lapses in attention slowed working memory, slowed duration of thought, and blunted mood.[15]

Instead of resolving to the negatives of sleep deprivation, we should look to the science of sleep hygiene. We need to learn ways to minimize the damage of sleep deprivation or impairment. Whenever sleep is in limited quantity, some of the harm is corrected with quality. One example is to find the time and place to take a power nap of 15 to 20 minutes in the middle of the day. Sleep improvement looks different for each individual surgeon. It is critical to develop a personal routine that works for you. Maybe you are a person who has an early clinic day start, but you like to sleep in. One solution is to start clinic day a little later and finish the clinic day later if that allows you to get improved quality of sleep.

Nutrition

When it comes to discussions about nutrition or diet, most orthopedic surgeons probably start to tune out. We either think that our constant activity can metabolize everything or we simply do not care. When pressed, we generally know to avoid fatty foods and excessive calories. However, the challenges are usually the availability of healthy choices or even any food at all. Early starts and long workdays with increasing inefficiencies often lead us to just want to get our cases done. Clinic days are usually no better. On-call days are even more difficult to make good choices when working into the night. The snacks available in most surgeon's lounges or hospital cafeterias are not as healthy, and fast food is often the most available on the way into the hospital for an urgent case.

Unfortunately, there is almost no data within the surgical literature on diet or nutrition and its relationship to well-being for surgeons. High-performance athletes have paid much more attention in recent years to the impact of nutrition on optimal performance. Most surgeons would agree that many of the demands of our career make us high-performance athletes. Whether it be appropriate hydration, healthy intake and portions, or the avoidance of unhealthy intake and portions, the science of nutrition also continues to advance. Healthy and unhealthy eating habits are particularly relevant to diet success and failure.

Surgeons often find it difficult to maintain healthy and consistent eating schedules. When you operate all day, sometimes you do not have time for breakfast, lunch, or dinner. Think about the things you can do to improve your diet. Set your nutrition goals. Create a proactive plan. Consider a simple strategy of gradually eliminating or adjusting one unhealthy eating habit at a time and/or increasing or adjusting one healthy habit at a time. One of the most common barriers to success is the distraction of any small failure that distracts from the implementation and follow through of the nutrition plan. Expect small failures. Maintain the intent. Immediately recommit to the plan. As you build your momentum from small successes, you have a greater chance of building that positive mindset that allows one to make healthier choices over time. It is important to remember that perfection is not the goal. Just getting a little better over time is the real goal.

Injury Prevention

One would think that orthopedic surgeons would be particularly focused on the musculo-skeletal injuries from work-related overuse that many of our patients present with. But the culture of orthopedic surgery and the personality of orthopedic surgeons sustains self-sacrifice at significant surgeon expense. Most surgeons would rather just get the surgery done quickly. As long as the outcome for the patient is great, we would rather not take the small amounts of time that are necessary to adjust our body, the table, or the equipment. The act of performing

any type of surgery is strenuous and is a known cause and exacerbation of musculoskeletal strain and injuries.[16] Some operations in orthopedic surgery require greater forces and are physically demanding on the surgeon, such as intramedullary nail extraction, reducing a dislocated hip or shoulder, and some fracture reductions. Within orthopedic surgery there is limited literature detailing this specific subject, and there is low awareness of ergonomics.[17]

Ergonomics is defined as the study of design and arrangement of things people use so as to optimize efficiency. It also deals with the prevention and management of occupational injury. According to the Occupational Safety and Health Administration, "an occupational injury is any wound or damage of the body resulting from an event in the work environment."[18] Although acute strains occur and "heal," the cumulative injuries sustained during the course of a successful orthopedic career ultimately cause a disability, nagging injury that decreases surgery efficiency or can lead to early retirement.[19] Causes are numerous and attributed to static forces during surgery, positioning of the surgeon, positioning of the patient, and operative surgical approach. Body parts most affected included upper extremities, spine, and generalized muscle pain. In one study, only 30% of surgeons stated that they purposefully enacted a specific plan to help improve ergonomics, and the same study found that only 30% of surgeons polled received medical care for their ailments.[19] Ergonomic improvement modalities include adjusting table height for maximum efficiency, using antifatigue mats during surgery, and intraoperative microbreaks. Proposed in a study for general surgeons are targeted stretching microbreaks for 90 seconds every 20 to 40 minutes while maintaining sterile technique to include stretching of neck flexion, extension, and lateral rotation; backward shoulder rolls with chest stretch; upper back and hand stretch; low back flexion and extension with gluteus maximus squeezes; and forefoot and heel lifts for lower extremity and ankle stretches. Fifty-seven percent of study participants reported improvement of their physical performance and 38% reported improved mental focus. Surgeons also reported decreased pain scores after surgeries that included microbreaks. Long-term benefits were not investigated.[20] Another study recommended that operating table height should be at a height where the top of a patient is at waist level to the surgeon.[21]

Not instituting ergonomic considerations early in one's practice is dangerous, and the result may have a compounding effect over one's career. Take 5 minutes to improve your ergonomic efficiency and it may well add 5 years to your career as a surgeon. The immediate benefits can also be seen in decreased surgeon pain scores following operations.

MENTAL WELLNESS

Orthopedic surgeons are intelligent and knowledgeable. Most of us pride ourselves in what we know. Adult learning theory research demonstrates that we all learn differently. Some of us have achieved our intellectual success through learning growth strategies, whereas others have used more negative strategies. Depending on our internal and external drivers, surgeons may respond with healthy resilience or wellness versus perfectionism, "imposter syndrome," and other internal challenges to our mental well-being. Our current training system and health care environment uses many strategies of negative resilience training, such as shaming, blaming, guilting, and pimping. The challenges are that we are exposed to a different mixture of internal and external negative drivers to acute and chronic mental injury. Everyone wants the ideal solution, and that too is different for each surgeon and each organization or team.

Issues creating mental distress range from administrative burdens, fighting for insurance authorizations, electronic medical record charting, experiencing adverse patient outcomes, and malpractice lawsuits. Depending on the quantity of these mental stressors and the quantity of mental wellness recovery, the effects on individual surgeons is different. For example, the number one stressor for most physicians is frequently the electronic medical record. Some estimates are that it takes physicians 2 hours of time on an electronic medical record for every hour of face-to-face patient time and that many physicians have to use "pajama time" after their children go to bed to complete charting responsibilities. In essence, any dissatisfying activity has the potential to wear down resilience, and vice versa.

Acute mental stress has been shown to impair complex cognitive functions, decision making, and team performance. One study showed that acute stress and performance during surgery were inversely proportional and significant. The authors of the same study also believe the inverse stress-surgical performance relationship is more pronounced than the findings in their article.[22] Mental distress is cumulative and leads to poor outcomes, such as relationship problems, divorce, substance or alcohol abuse, depression, anxiety, post-traumatic stress disorder (PTSD), and suicide. Up to 6.8% of physicians have alcohol dependence issues,[23] and up to 33% of surgeons have had divorces.[24] Although depression incidence is similar to non–health care populations, suicide mortality among physicians is much higher than other professionals: a male physician's risk of mortality is 1.5 to 3.8 times higher, whereas a female physician's risk is 3.7 to 4.5 times higher.[25,26] It should be chilling to all physicians that up to 1 in 16 surgeons have considered suicide.[27] Secondary traumatic stress, which occurs after repeated or extreme stress of patients that one is taking care of, is known to occur in up to 80% of physicians taking care of trauma patients. Although also being the effect of cumulative stresses, secondary traumatic stress can manifest over a longer duration with signs mirroring that of acute mental stress, such as impaired decision making.[28]

Solutions for mental wellness are analogous to physical wellness: prevention through constructive exercises of mental health combined with recovery or management of acute and chronic mental injuries. If we learn to recover and grow from these mental injuries, we can improve our mental resilience in sustainable ways. Perception is a key component of mental stress and a more difficult transition. Research clearly shows that high performers grow from stress and anxiety that we perceive is valuable to our learning and growth, whereas stress that is perceived as interfering with growth and learning is distress.

Visualization

An often underused mental tool for decreasing the perception of stress is visualization. Often used by elite athletes (and some surgeons) one mentally rehearses an action or event without physically doing it. A surgical procedure can be mentally rehearsed the night before a complex operation, which can help anticipate challenges and subsequently decrease the perceived stress. Studies have shown that this mental practice enhances performance and cognitive skills.[29] Visualization can also be used in any other context that requires mental preparation, such as preparing for a difficult conversation or public speaking.

Meditation and Mindfulness

Although many orthopedic surgeons think meditation and mindfulness are the fluffy stuff, these mental exercises are incredibly effective for injury prevention and managing acute and chronic mental injury. Meditation and many other mindfulness exercises are defined as a habitual process of training one's mind to focus and redirect thoughts. The exercise usually focuses one or more of our senses during the process, which can be breaths, physical sensations, or repetition of words or phrases that evoke relaxation of the mind. Studies have shown some forms of meditation to decrease stress and serum cortisol levels.[30] Depending on the type of meditation performed, studies have shown hypertrophy in cortical thickness of the brain in meditation practitioners, in areas varying depending on the type of meditation being practiced.[31] Studies have shown that an extensive time commitment is not necessary for statistically significant benefits from meditation.[32] Like any physical exercise and skill, mental exercise and skills can start small and grow at the individual surgeon's desire and time availability. Initial time commitments can be as little as 30 to 60 seconds. The key is to practice consistently to see the benefit in the longer term. Deliberate practice results in faster and greater improvements.

Resiliency Training

The overlap between physical, mental, emotional, and spiritual wellness is significant. Often this is packaged into the concept of stress management, mental toughness, or resiliency training. Because graduating from medical school, residency, and often fellowship can feel like completing some of the most intense military training programs, orthopedic surgeons often do not like the suggestion that they are not already tremendously resilient or able to handle almost any stress. In fact, they are and can. However, we hypothesize that the most effective resiliency training programs require unlearning some of the negative drivers of resilience and emphasize learning ways to positively affect our perception. Effective resiliency training programs are also growth oriented and allow customization by the individual learner. Usually lasting several weeks and a moderate time commitment, resiliency training is courselike in that one outlines and applies principles to better adapt to stress, maintain positivity, and become more flexible with the unknown. However, a large time commitment is not always required. One successful program found benefits with resiliency, perceived stress, anxiety, and overall quality of life at 8 weeks with just a few sessions with a time commitment of fewer than 2 hours per session.[33]

EMOTIONAL WELLNESS

Orthopedic surgeons are not particularly well trained in emotional wellness. No matter the difficult emotion, such as anger, frustration, sadness, anxiety, or jealousy, they are taught to hide it or "suck it up." Although some orthopedic surgeons are emotionally intelligent, these skills are not necessarily enhanced within our training and health care environment. In fact, many unhealthy strategies, poor emotional regulation, or negative coping strategies are modeled, encouraged, and rewarded. Our workplace is not only physically hazardous but emotionally hazardous too. Our patients and their family members are dealing with the unfamiliar and the emotionally challenging times of illness or injury. When empathy is unchecked, we expose ourselves to this emotional trauma vicariously. Our physical and mental exhaustion can further worsen our ability to self-regulate our emotions. We can become acutely or chronically emotionally exhausted. Cynicism, the objectification of people and colleagues, leads to detachment or the opposite of healthy engagement. These are two of the three key components of burnout, if their frequency is too high.

As in other specialties, high-stress situations and repetitive crises can also take an emotional toll on an orthopedic surgeon. A surgeon wishes to use one's skills to positively affect a patient outcome and help them heal, but complications happen to everyone. Patient complications can be especially difficult for a surgeon to deal with and may linger long after a complication has occurred. The effects on the surgeon of complications that are not processed also seem to be cumulative and can eventually lead to PTSD and decreased emotional wellness.[34] PTSD and secondary traumatic stress can be aggravated or sustained by denial and avoidance coping. In addition to a complication being potentially devastating to a surgeon's psyche, litigation may follow, whether warranted or not. Some surgeons learn from complications and are better able to provide care, but others become risk-averse, especially after a poor medicolegal case or outcome, developing practices that focus on decreasing the risk of a lawsuit instead of what is best for the patient.[34] The repetitive effects of these emotional challenges can also decrease productivity and enthusiasm at work, increase the risk of medical errors, and increase risk of ruining personal relationships outside of work. Emotional isolation, defined as the absence of a close communicator or confidant, can have enormous implications. Surgeons are at significant risk for emotional loneliness because they are largely self-reliant, have a drive for ever-increasing success, and as a group have poor emotional connections throughout the field.[35] A step that most surgeons can take is to reach and talk more with colleagues to decrease any isolation.

Emotional wellness involves the development of strength, flexibility, balance, and conditioning of the emotional "muscle." Similar to physical and mental wellness strategies, we can prevent some emotional injury through growing our emotional intelligence. Emotional rest and recovery or management of acute and chronic emotional injuries can come from many practices including cognitive reframing, self-compassion, peer support, community, and connection.

Emotional Intelligence

Although IQ is thought to be largely static, emotional intelligence is largely defined by parameters that have much more potential to expand from emotional skill training. Orthopedic surgeons can cultivate the following:

1. Motivation: the passion in work for internal rather than external reasons.
2. Empathy: bedside manner and ability to understand the emotions of others.
3. Self-awareness: the ability to recognize their own strengths, weaknesses, moods, emotions, and motivations and their effect on others.
4. Self-regulation: the ability to realistically self-assess, control, and redirect disruptive impulses and moods.
5. Social skills: team building and proficiency in managing relationships, finding common ground with others, and building rapport.

Residency programs have recognized that emotional intelligence is an important component of success in training, because one study found a deficiency of emotional intelligence in orthopedic residents.[36] Opportunities for advancing these skills take only a little bit of investigating.

Cognitive Reframing

A first step in maintaining a strong emotional awareness is cultivating an optimistic attitude. There are optimistic colleagues within our field, and we would benefit from recognizing how they function among us. A skill that they often possess is the ability to see opportunity in challenge. The more challenging the environment and the emotional response, the more difficult it is for most of us to remain optimistic. Cognitive reframing is a technique within cognitive behavioral therapy that has shown success in managing these challenges.[37] Although perhaps oversimplified, cognitive reframing involves the skill of taking our reactive negative thoughts and balancing them with more rational, wiser, more positive, more hopeful thoughts that can lead to changes in our endocrine response and action or behaviors that are more desirable. We mindfully reframe the reactive negative irrational thought to an intentional positive rational thought. For example, staying late one evening to complete an urgent fracture repair can be viewed as an opportunity to positively impact a person as opposed to the negative view of missing time at home with family in the evening.

Self-Compassion

We believe that orthopedic surgeons have a greater capacity for learning empathy and compassion for others, because these characteristics often led them into a career in medicine. However, positive self-talk is not taught to and rarely demonstrated by orthopedic surgeons that we are aware of. Self-compassion, as defined by Neff and Germer,[38] is "being touched by one's own suffering." This ultimately leads to "treating oneself with compassion and concern." The three tenants of self-compassion are:

1. Increasing self-awareness and honesty with oneself
2. Allowing self-acceptance
3. Accepting the "human condition" that people are imperfect

When one begins to practice self-compassion, it is then possible to learn to cope with one's flaws as a normal exercise of human nature. This allows a person to learn from any experience, whether positive or negative, and deal with issues in a way that avoids self-degradation or overrumination.[38] Self-compassion is a mindfulness exercise. When applied, the practice of self-compassion has shown to consistently improve one's overall wellness; decrease stressful responses to stressful stimuli; and allow positive improvements in psychological strengths, relationships, and emotional intelligence.[39] The only thing a person can control is their reaction to any situation. Self-compassion and mindfulness allow one to better regulate that reaction.

SPIRITUAL WELLNESS

Spiritual wellness is the most personal of all the components of wellness and takes into account one's values, beliefs, and purposes. Although the degree of protection provided is not known, genuine spirituality correlates with decreased rates of burnout in physicians. A decreased sense of personal accomplishment, the third measure of burnout in the Maslach Burnout Inventory, should be a self-assessment of our achievements within purpose. However, being accomplished is also impacted by our perception of external assessments, mostly culturally based. When our values, beliefs, or purposes conflict with society, organizations, and/or the health care cultural norms, this conflict causes moral and spiritual injury. The concept of moral injury has resonated much better with physicians than the term "burnout" ever since a 2018 article by Dean and coworkers.[40] They argue "without understanding the critical difference between burnout and moral injury, the wounds will never heal and physicians and patients alike will continue to suffer the consequences." Their article has done a great job in initiating conversations and offering solutions, and it is hoped directing additional research into these areas.

Dean and coworkers[40] propose leadership (and perhaps regulatory changes) that can minimize the moral injury to physicians from "the death by a thousand cuts" of electronic medical records, administrative burdens, and competing business demands versus patient care.[40] Each of these are significant drivers to an unhealthy spirit in orthopedic surgeons, because they require physicians to do menial tasks that also often contradict their purpose in practicing medicine, caring for patients with quality, compassion, and great knowledge. Most of us would have no difficulty in creating a list of complaints or things for which we are ungrateful.

More severe moral injury comes from activities directly in line with our purpose but which have the opposite result, such as adverse outcomes, litigation, and misunderstandings with patients, their families, and many others. Spiritual injury can come from our competitive nature, egos, and other values or beliefs that become too extreme, such as perfectionism, martyrdom, superheroism, and just "sucking it up" for everything that contradicts our morals, values, and beliefs. The consequence of moral and spiritual injury is the premature departure of many talented, knowledgeable, and passionate surgeons from clinical careers and leadership within the field. Far worse, alone or in combination with the other components of wellness, it can lead to physician suicide; mental illness; or complete loss of values, beliefs, and purpose. What are we organizationally and culturally willing to take responsibility for in orthopedic surgery? Perhaps our collective values and beliefs, and other "cultural" biases within orthopedic surgery contribute to the eating of our own and the avoidance of others from entering this amazingly rewarding career, including those with racial, gender, and other human diversity.

As we have already argued, surgeon wellness is about addressing all of these components, rather than just one. We acknowledge that spiritual wellness is important, but to our knowledge values, beliefs, and purpose have not been well studied. One study on medical students and burnout defined spirituality using the National Institutes of Health definition "Having to do with deep, often religious, feelings and beliefs, including a person's sense of peace, purpose, connection to others, and beliefs about the meaning of life." One study showed that 55% of physicians believe that their religious beliefs influence their practice of medicine.[41]

Simply reading the few articles on professional satisfaction within orthopedic surgery highlights some of the inherent biases in the research. If we leverage what we know in the other three components of wellness, we could hypothesize that by better aligning our values, beliefs, and purpose to what we do, then we could strengthen our spiritual resilience, allow for spiritual rest and recovery, and lessen the consequences of acute or chronic moral injury through hobbies or joys outside of work, sabbaticals, medical missions, job changes, and engaging in simple healthy spiritual practices.

Passion and Purpose

Why do we do what we do? Why did we go into orthopedic surgery in the first place? What would reinvigorate our professional purpose? What is one's purpose with respect to our patients? Spiritual wellness is thought of as a person's values and ideals that cultivate purpose and provide meaning to life. The purpose can be one's direction in life, a tool that one uses from a higher power to improve other's lives, or a belief of a path a high power sets for an individual. Spirituality is faith-based or nonreligious. Addressing our passion and purpose is internally disruptive if we find ourselves misaligned. Be forgiving to yourself and others. Have faith that even our purpose can be improved. Simply reflect without undue pressure. Begin activities that bring more joy or alignment with your values and beliefs. Say no or phase out activities that conflict with purpose and passion.

We would be remiss to leave out a traditional and effective passion and purpose of being the best at what we do and maintaining high standards for the care that we provide our patients. But it is important to point out that perfectionism can easily sap passion and purpose. Excellence and perfection are not synonymous. Excellence connotes that we can all get a little bit better, no matter our skill level. Perfection is not attainable by anyone, even the truly elite. Blend this passion for performance improvement with the understanding that there are many obstacles in our current health care system to achieving excellence as often as we would like, add in some other supportive purpose, and you just might find sustainable spiritual wellness.

Gratitude

The reactive brain by default places greater emphasis on challenges and the negatives of life, which steer us to survival and other innate drives. If we want to override this part of the brain with higher reasoning and opposing endorphins, we can create that process. Creating a practice of gratitude is one way to balance out to a more positive rational brain. What are we thankful for? What simple list can you create to acknowledge a few things for which we are grateful? Creating focus on and appreciation for the good things in our careers and lives rebuilds the positive spirit. Gratitude also helps us raise awareness of our values, beliefs, and purpose and gives thanks to those around us. One way or another develop a gratitude practice that is much more frequent than yearly holidays or occasional events. Daily is recommended.

BROADER STRATEGIES TO IMPROVE ALL COMPONENTS OF WELLNESS

Community and Connection

Human beings are a "herd species" that thrive on input from one another. Emotional loneliness has physical manifestations, such as increases in cardiovascular disease, anxiety, depression, and decreases cognitive functions. All of this leads to increased workplace stress.[35] To oppose emotional (and mental) isolation, even orthopedic surgeons have sought connection to others through community, organizations, clubs, and educational conferences. Positive social interactions have a known mechanism of increasing oxytocin, and fighting stress and

building trust among its participants.[42,43] Finding community and acceptance within a workplace (or even outside of the workplace) can greatly reduce emotional loneliness. Interacting with others who help you process your thoughts and emotions in healthy ways rather than keeping you in a negative frame of mind is a tremendous boost to your emotional well-being. Have caution in the social media realm or groups where wellness is not encouraged or negativity is too common. Look for connection and communities that support your wellness goals, that is, cycling group, weight loss, stress reduction, and improved resiliency. Camaraderie with other physicians and professionals who share your challenges, ideal values, and beliefs can improve spiritual wellness.

Peer Support

Having a close confidant, mentor, or peer group where one receives active listening, constructive feedback, and acknowledgment in a supportive and safe environment to share clinical and life experiences enhances our growth. Facilitated peer groups with regularly scheduled group meetings has shown benefit for residents and attending physicians in some surgeon wellness programs.[44] When set up for physician peers of similar experience, not remedial, and participation encouraged, peer support groups are effective in processing the usual challenges of being an orthopedic surgeon.

Professional Coaching

Professional coaching, also known as executive coaching or life coaching, is a partnering with clients in a thought-provoking and creative process that inspires them to maximize their personal and professional potential.[45] Coaching has shown to be an effective remedy for decreasing emotional exhaustion, increasing operative efficiency, and decreasing symptoms of burnout.[46] Additionally, reported benefits include greater positivity; better, longer focus; and graduating self-directed improvement. Coaching benefits are seen in less than 1 hour of coaching per month.[47,48] Overall, coaching is still in the early stages but looks to be a strong physician wellness tenant. Professional coaching helps the client find their own solutions to their own challenges. It is important to remember that coaching is a different approach from mentoring, where advice is handed down from one person in authority to one who is seeking advice and a similar career path. Coaching can be received in any or all of the areas of surgeon wellness.

Organizational and Cultural Change

Our article focuses on wellness strategies that orthopedic surgeons can address individually or with peers, mentors, or coaches. According to most researchers, 80% to 90% of the drivers of burnout, lack of professional satisfaction, and unwellness comes from poorly designed or punitive institutional regulations that appropriately address patient outcomes, value in health care delivery, and patient satisfaction but without any attention to physician satisfaction or wellness. It would be another article topic to focus on the systemic or organizational changes that could positively affect physician wellness. Attention to physician satisfaction, fulfillment, experience, and wellness and high-quality, efficient patient care is considered the "quadruple aim." We strongly encourage leaders within our organizations to make this a priority with the appropriate budget, infrastructure, resources, and time. Rates of physician burnout would be drastically decreased with optimization of individual and institutional protective factors.[49,50]

SUMMARY: PRACTICING WELLNESS

Surgeons are often trained to be lone rangers working in isolation. This can often lead to diminished wellness and burnout. In each of the wellness components discussed in this article (physical, mental, emotional, and spiritual), there are concepts and solutions that can help us improve and maintain our overall wellness. We have mentioned numerous examples, but at the end of the day it is up to each individual surgeon to determine what works best for them. Make a conscious effort to improve your wellness in any way you can. No one can master all four wellness components overnight, but everyone can improve in some way. Start small and take baby steps. The most important thing is to be proactive and consistent. In order for one to maintain wellness, one has to practice wellness habits. Over time, you will see the fruits of your labors!

CLINICS CARE POINTS

- Maintain the physical foundation with healthier eating and sleep habits, a regular exercise regimen that includes strengthening, stretching, and cardio, and attention to ergonomics for injury prevention.
- Train the mental circuitry with meditation, mindfulness, visualization, and other forms of resilience training.
- Sustain emotional well-being through self-compassion, cognitive reframing, and emotional intelligence training.
- Obtain or regain spiritual health by allowing practices of gratitude, analysis of passion and purpose, and embracing excellence while rejecting perfectionism.
- Entertain community / connection, peer support, professional coaching, and organizational / cultural change as a means to achieve your fullest potential.

DISCLOSURE

Dr J.M. Smith owns and operates www.surgeonmasters.com, where he is the managing partner and works as a surgeon coach and trains others in physician coaching. Dr E.A. Boe has no disclosures. Dr R. Will has no disclosures.

REFERENCES

1. Jager AJ, Tuty MA, Kao AC. Association between physician burnout and identification with medicine as a calling. Mayo Clin Proc 2017;92(3): 415–22.
2. Kane L. "Medscape national physician burnout & suicide report 2020: the generational divide." medscape 2020. Available at: www.medscape.com/slideshow/2020-lifestyle-burnout-6012460. Accessed June 15, 2020.
3. Balch CM, Freischlag JA, Shanafelt TD. Stress and burnout among surgeons: understanding and managing the syndrome and avoiding the adverse consequences. Arch Surg 2009;144(4):371–6.
4. Centers for Disease Control and Prevention. Physical activity for everyone. Available at: www.cdc.gov/physicalactivity/everyone/guidelines/adults.html#aerobic. Accessed May 12, 2020.
5. Maddeus M. The resilience bank account: skills for optimal performance. Ann Thorac Surg 2020;109(1): 18–25.
6. Tari AR, Norevik CS, Scrimgeour NR, et al. Are the neuroprotective effects of exercise training systemically mediated? Prog Cardiovasc Dis 2019;62: 94–101.
7. Pederson BK. Physical activity and muscle-brain crosstalk. Nat Rev Endocrinol 2019;15:383–92.
8. Voss MW, Nagamatsu LS, Liu-Ambrose, et al. Exercise, brain, and cognition across the life span. J Appl Phys 2011;111:1505–13.
9. Cotman CW, Berchtold NC. Exercise: a behavioral intervention to enhance brain health and plasticity. Trends Neurosci 2002;25:295–301.
10. Basso JC, Suzuki WA. The effects of acute exercise on mood, cognition, neurophysiology, and neurochemical pathways: a review. Brain Plast 2017;2:127–52.

11. Watson NF, Badr MF, Belenky G, et al. Joint consensus statement of the American Academy of Sleep Medicine and Sleep Research Society on the recommended amount of sleep for a healthy adult: methodology and discussion. Sleep 2015; 38(8):1161–83.

12. Naiman R. Dreamless: the silent epidemic of REM sleep loss. Ann N Y Acad Sci 2017;1406:77–85.

13. Cappuccio FP, D'Elia L, Strazzullo P, et al. Sleep duration and all-cause mortality: a systematic review and meta-analysis of prospective studies. Sleep 2010;33:585–92.

14. Iftikhar IH, Donley MA, Mindel J, et al. Sleep duration and metabolic syndrome, an updated dose-risk metaanalysis. Ann Am Thorac Soc 2015;12: 1364–72.

15. Banks S, Dinges DF. Behavioral and physiological consequences of sleep restriction. J Clin Sleep Med 2007;3(5):519–28.

16. Buckle PW, Devereux JJ. The nature of work-related neck and upper limb musculoskeletal disorders. Appl Ergon 2002;33(3):207–17.

17. Davis WT, Sathiyakumar V, Jahangir AA, et al. Occupational injury among orthopedic surgeons. J Bone Joint Surg Am 2013;95(1–6):e107.

18. Bureau of Labor Statistics. Occupational safety and health definitions. Available at: http://www.bls.gov/iif/oshdef.htm. Accessed May 31, 2020.

19. Stucky CH, Cromwell KD, Voss RK, et al. Surgeon symptoms, strain, and selections: systematic review and meta-analysis of surgical ergonomics. Ann Med Surg (Lond) 2018;27:1–8.

20. Park AE, Zahiri HR, Hallbeck MS, et al. Intraoperative "micro breaks" with targeted stretching enhance surgeon physical function and mental focus: a multicenter cohort study. Ann Surg 2017; 265(2):340–6.

21. Wohl DL, Hubbard T. Physician safety is patient safety: good surgical ergonomics to optimize patient care. ENTnet.org Bulletin 2019;38(3):14–5.

22. Grantcharov PD, Boillat T, Elkabany S, et al. Acute mental stress and surgical performance. BJS Open 2019;3(1):119–25.

23. Kuerer HM, Eberlein TJ, Pollock RE, et al. Career satisfaction, practice patterns and burnout among surgical oncologists: report on the quality of life of members of the society of surgical oncology. Ann Surg Oncol 2007;14(11):3043–53.

24. Rollman BL, Mead LA, Wang NY. Medical specialty and the incidence of divorce. N Engl J Med 1997; 336(11):800–3.

25. Center C, Davis M, Detre T, et al. Confronting depression and suicide in physicians: a consensus statement. JAMA 2003;289(23):3161–6.

26. Lindeman S, Laara E, Hakko H, et al. A systematic review on gender-specific suicide mortality in medical doctors. Br J Psychiatry 1996;168(3): 274–9.

27. Shanafelt TD, Balch CM, Dyrbye L, et al. Special report: suicidal ideation among American surgeons. Arch Surg 2011;146:5462.

28. Teel J, Reynolds M, Bennett M, et al. Secondary traumatic stress among physiatrists treating trauma patients. Proc (Bayl Univ Med Cent) 2019;32(2): 209–14.

29. Arora S, Aggarwal R, Moran A, et al. Mental practice: effective stress management training for novice surgeons. J Am Coll Surg 2011;212(2): 225–33.

30. Engert V, Kok BE, Papassotiriou I. Specific reduction in cortisol stress reactivity after social but not attention-based mental training. Sci Adv 2017;3: e1700495.

31. Singer T, Engert V. It matters what you practice: differential training effects on subjective experience, behavior, brain and body in the resource project. Curr Opin Psychol 2018;28:151–8.

32. Basso JC, McHale A, Ende V. Brief, daily meditation enhances attention, memory, mood, and emotional regulation in non-experienced meditators. Behav Brain Res 2019;356:208–20.

33. Sood A, Prasad K, Schroeder D, et al. Stress management and resilience training among department of medicine faculty: a pilot randomized clinical trial. J Gen Intern Med 2011;26(8): 858–61.

34. Sirnivasa S, Gurney J, Koea J. Potential consequences of patient complications for surgeon well-being: a systematic review. JAMA Surg 2019; 154(5):451–7.

35. Masi CM, Chen H, Hawkley LC. A meta-analysis of interventions to reduce loneliness. Pers Soc Psychol Rev 2011;15:219–66.

36. Chan K, Petrisor B, Bhandari M. Emotional intelligence in orthopedic surgery residents. Can J Surg 2014;57:89–93.

37. Allespach H, Diaz Y, Burg MA, et al. Daily self-care and cognitive restructuring: a potentially potent prescription for physician wellness. Cogent Med 2019;6(1):1704151.

38. Neff KD, Germer CK. A pilot study and randomized controlled trial of the mindful self-compassion program. J Clin Psychol 2013;69:28–44.

39. Neff KD, Pommier E. The relationship between self-compassion and other-focused concern among college undergraduates, community adults, and practicing meditators. Self Identity 2012. https://doi.org/10.1080/15298868.2011. 649546.

40. Dean W, Talbot S, Dean A. Reframing clinician distress: moral injury not burnout. Fed Pract 2019; 36(9):400–2.

41. Curlin FA, Lantos JD, Roach CJ, et al. Religious characteristics of U.S. physicians: a national survey. J Gen Intern Med 2005;20(7):629–34.

42. Glaser JE, Glaser RD. The neurochemistry of positive conversations. Harv Bus Rev 2014. Available at: https://hbr.org/2014/06/the-neurochemistry-of-positive-conversations.

43. Bussing A, Janko A, Baumann K, et al. Spiritual needs among patients with chronic pain diseases and cancer living in a secular society. Pain Med 2013;14(9):1362–73.

44. Mueller CM, Buckle M, Post L. A facilitated-group approach to wellness in surgical residency. JAMA Surg 2018;153(11):1043–4.

45. International Coaching Federation. Available at: https://coachfederation.org/. Accessed June 01, 2020.

46. Gazelle G, Liebschutz JM, Riess H. Physician burnout: coaching a way out. J Gen Intern Med 2015;30(4):508–13.

47. Smith JM. Surgeon coaching: why and how. J Pediatr Orthop 2020;40(Suppl 1):S33–7.

48. Dyrbye L, Shanafelt T, Gill P, et al. Effect of a professional coaching intervention on the well-being and distress of physicians: a pilot randomized clinical trial. JAMA Intern Med 2019;179(10):1406–14.

49. Sargent MC, Sotile W, Sotile MO, et al. Quality of life during orthopaedic training and academic practice: Part 1. Orthopaedic surgery residents and faculty. J Bone Joint Surg Am 2009;91(10):2395–405.

50. Saleh KJ, Quick JC, Conaway M, et al. The prevalence and severity of burnout among academic orthopaedic departmental leaders. J Bone Joint Surg Am 2007;89(4):896–903.

Life Long Learning
The Attending and Educator in Orthopedic Trauma

Clay A. Spitler, MD

KEYWORDS
• Orthopedic trauma • Adult education • Resilience

KEY POINTS
• Since its inception, surgical training has drawn on an apprenticeship model, where the progressive transfer of knowledge, responsibility, and autonomy to a trainee occurs over time as they work side by side with experienced physicians.
• In most residency programs, fracture care and orthopedic trauma comprises 8 to 12 months of most 5-year programs.
• For many reasons, training programs are shifting towards competency-based learning in order to ensure the quality of trainees produced.
• The "hidden curriculum" includes the attitudes and behaviors that educators model for trainees. As our trainees learn to be orthopaedic surgeons, they will carry the behaviors and attitudes learned via the hidden curriculum into practice.

GOALS/OBJECTIVES

As orthopedic surgeons, our formal education begins when we are around 5 years old, and in most cases, continues in a structured way until the fourth decade of life. This formal education is the basis of our medical knowledge and is critical to our success as physicians, but it is not the only type of knowledge that is essential to becoming a well-rounded physician educator. Our personalities, family upbringing, and environments shape how we think and interact with those around us. Together these tools, traits, and surroundings shape our mindset and it is this mindset that helps set the course of our lives.

A growth mindset can loosely be described as one that views every part of our lives as having the capacity for improvement or malleability. This mindset is an important lens through which we can view our lives, respond to failures, and celebrate our achievements. This foundational attitude allows us to learn from our shortcomings and improve on them, remain humble in success, and to continue our daily pursuit of excellence with dogged determination. As an educator, our learners can memorize the didactic curriculum we provide to them, but the "hidden curriculum" that we model to them is what they emulate after they leave our training programs.[1]

What Is the Goal of Orthopedic Trauma Surgery?

The goal of orthopedic trauma surgery is to provide excellent care to patients who have sustained traumatic injuries. In high-functioning systems, this is accomplished in conjunction with general trauma surgeons, critical care physicians, emergency room physicians, and medicine/geriatric physicians. This team approach is needed with other services and within our own groups to be able to achieve optimal outcomes. On an individual basis, it requires that we are compassionate and caring with each individual

Department of Orthopaedics, University of Alabama at Birmingham, 510 20th Street South, Faculty Office Tower 901, Birmingham, AL 35294, USA
E-mail address: caspitler@uabmc.edu

Orthop Clin N Am 52 (2021) 53–59
https://doi.org/10.1016/j.ocl.2020.09.001
0030-5898/21/© 2020 Elsevier Inc. All rights reserved.

patient and take their circumstances into account as we formulate our plan for their treatment. It requires of us, foresight and technical skill to effectively plan and execute each fracture surgery to provide the best possible outcome for our patients. It also requires attention to detail and empathy as we help these patients rehabilitate their injuries. At the group level, this requires a team-based approach that relies on the strengths of each member of the team and a level of trust within the team to function at its most optimal level.

What Is the Goal of an Orthopedic Educator?

The goal of an orthopedic educator is to pass on necessary knowledge and technical skills to those we work alongside in the process of caring for patients with traumatic injuries. Those most commonly associated with this education are residents and fellows, but also include physician assistants, nurse practitioners, radiology technicians, nurses, physical therapists, and other physician colleagues. Each interaction requires tactful interpersonal skills to effectively communicate at an appropriate level with each person with whom we interact. Although constructive and respectful dialogue should always be used, methods of communication used with junior residents cannot and should not be used with emergency room or general surgery trauma attendings. The most effective manner of communication may vary by individual or position and is learned after repeated encounters. As an educator, we must continue to make every effort to stay abreast of the most current orthopedic literature, so we remain on the cutting edge in the way we educate our trainees. Teaching requires that we pass along accurate information and techniques, but also remain consistent in the way that we practice medicine and respectfully interact with those around us. The goal of an educator is to not only teach information, but also to pass on the important skill of "learning how to learn" so that we are all equipped to handle the changes that we will inevitably face.[2]

The good news is no one is perfect. No orthopedic surgeon, whether they are at the beginning of their career, nor the surgeon who has practiced for 30 years gets every single one of these things right every single time. In the book *Grit*, Angela Duckworth makes a distinction between talent, a natural affinity for a certain activity, and skill, which is the mastery that results from hours of intentional practice of that same activity, emphasizing that "without effort, talent is nothing more than your unmet

potential."[3] Being an effective lifelong learner requires self-awareness to identify our individual strengths and weaknesses, capitalize on our strengths, while working diligently to develop in the areas we need improvement. The mindset needed to be a successful lifelong learner requires a personal commitment to continual improvement. One of the foundational principles of lifelong learning is that it is impossible to fully equip learners in school and formal training. To continue to be relevant, successful, and effective, surgeons must continually enhance their knowledge and skills.[2] All of this begins with an honest introspection and inventory of ourselves.

INTROSPECTION

There are skills and traits that are critical to being successful in the roles of attending surgeon and educator. Because we all have different backgrounds and natural gifts, some parts of the job are more natural to some surgeons, but all is learned and practiced.

Commitment to Self-Improvement

Lifelong learning is based on the understanding that at every point in our lives and careers we have yet to achieve perfection. As a result, there are traits and skills that we can continue to improve. The most effective way to understand my strengths and weaknesses comes through the critical and objective assessment of myself and by those around me. Those who seek feedback from superiors, peers, and learners are most likely to identify weaknesses to be improved and recognize personal strengths that can be built on.

Humility

"Humility is the foundation of all the other virtues hence, in the soul in which this virtue does not exist there cannot be any other virtue except in mere appearance."[4]
—Augustine

Humility is often misunderstood as a lack of confidence, thinking poorly of yourself, or thinking that you have little to offer to those around you. True humility is grounded in understanding the inherent value of every person around us, whether they are a patient, a coworker, or a colleague. In the professional context, humility should be characterized as lacking arrogance and the self-recognition that there is always room for improvement. It is this mindset that allows us to continually seek to get better, while knowing that we can learn from those around us. "Humility is not thinking less of yourself, it is thinking of yourself less."[5] This "others-centered" approach is a powerful tool in motivating us to be better physicians. The humility of a leader can powerfully impact the relationships and performance of a team or business to improve the overall success of the team.[6] The understanding that "I have not 'arrived'," and there is always room for improvement serves as fuel for the fire of the lifelong learner.

Drive for Excellence

There are different ways to describe the inner drive for excellence, but there lies in all of us a desire to be the best at the things we choose to make our focus. This inner drive has been demonstrated in the sports world, the business world, and has applications in medical education. The late, great Kobe Bryant, described his Mamba Mentality as "a constant quest to be better today than you were yesterday."[7] To borrow from Six Sigma, in the business world, every part of our work should be consistently under examination so we can identify areas for improvement. I will always carry with me the advice of one of my mentors shortly after completing residency "Take advantage of the opportunities that you have earned, work hard, and be better than just good." This inner drive must be manifested by our focused effort to improve, because as Vince Lombardi astutely pointed out "the only place success comes before work is in the dictionary."

Resilience

There will be personal and professional setbacks that we encounter in our profession and whether we like it or not, these setbacks often occur in plain view of our trainees. The response that we model for them is always a large part of the "hidden curriculum" and provide an opportunity to demonstrate a growth mindset and practice resilience. It allows us to teach them to embrace hardship, because situations that challenge us are some of the best opportunities for growth and learning. Each problem/challenge we face (whether it is clinical, administrative, or personal) can be seen as an occasion to learn and practice problem solving skills and ultimately be better personally for having dealt with the problem.[8]

APPRENTICESHIP

Since its inception, surgical training has drawn on an apprenticeship model, where the progressive transfer of knowledge, responsibility, and autonomy to a trainee occurs over time as they work side by side with experienced physicians. As surgical education continues to evolve to include proficiency-based evaluations and surgical simulation, there are important parts of the apprenticeship model that must remain firmly entrenched in our training programs. This experiential learning is critical to trainees as they begin to forge their surgical skills and will never be completely replaced by surgical simulation. Although surgical repetitions are gained with surgical simulation, there is no way to simulate the skills needed to interact with patients or develop an all-encompassing approach to patient care. These "softer" skills are best learned by observing and walking alongside an experienced mentor. Every resident enters training with a developed notion of self and others, but they learn how to interact with other physicians, nurses, operating room (OR) personnel, and administrators by watching and replicating the example they see modeled for them. This responsibility should weigh heavily on us as we train future generations of surgeons.

One of the important soft skills that helps us be effective teachers and leaders is emotional intelligence.[9] Emotional intelligence is an understanding our own emotions, the emotions of others, and possessing the ability to influence the emotions of others. This skill allows us to manage the different personalities around us, adapt to changing work conditions, and generates good will and a team first attitude in those around us.[10,11] These outcomes produce success in our workplaces and classrooms. When we consistently demonstrate these qualities, our trainees will have an example to follow and replicate this success as they begin practice.

There are many pressures that have led to a shift away from the apprenticeship model, including restrictions in resident work hours and increased financial pressure for efficiency. This has led to increased focus on a competency-based assessment of learning and the use of surgical simulation.

Competency-Based Learning

In most residency programs, fracture care and orthopedic trauma comprises 8 to 12 months of most 5-year programs. As a result, we as orthopedic trauma faculty, have more exposure to residents than any other subspecialty and the skills gained under our direction are expected to translate to all other subspecialties. Training programs seek to graduate competent residents, but anyone who has watched a large number of residents can agree that some have a more natural affinity for some surgical skills. How do we then ensure each graduate has reached an adequate level of competency before graduation?

The era in which we practice includes the challenges of resident work hour restrictions, increasing regulatory oversight, and increased financial pressures. With this backdrop, our goal as educators remains to produce competent trainees. These challenges have led to an evolution in the way that we teach and evaluate residents and it is important that we continue to evolve these processes to keep pace with the demands of our environment. Standardization of curricula and rotation schedules across all residency training programs is not possible for myriad reasons, but specific core surgical competencies can be identified and standardized. For example, to ensure that regardless of subspecialty training and location of residency program, graduating surgeons are able to adequately perform open reduction and internal fixation of an ankle or hip fracture and have met a standard set by a governing body (eg, Accreditation Council for Graduate Medical Education, American Board of Orthopaedic Surgery).

The setting of objective standards is necessary to ensure the quality of the training we provide, but we must also remind ourselves that one of the most important qualities that we can teach our trainees is the necessity of continuing to learn after the completion of formal training. Within the narrow field of orthopedic trauma surgery, current surgical techniques and their basic science underpinnings continue to evolve. Although I have practiced for what seems like a few short years, there are techniques that I consider a routine part of my practice today that I did not see in my residency (eg, dual plating or nail/plate for some distal femur fracture, induced membrane bone grafting). The rapidly changing nature of the field necessitates lifelong learning to provide state-of-the-art care for our patients throughout the entirety of our careers. If I fail to continue learning throughout my career, the field will pass me by, but engaging in the process of lifelong learning allows us to stand on the shoulders of the giants who have come before us, learn from our peers, and continue to push our field ahead.

Surgical Simulation

Although simulation in many orthopedic subspecialties remains in its infancy, it has been a part of the airline industry for more than 100 years and will continue to play an increasingly important role in orthopedic training going forward.

Mastery of any topic requires deliberate practice. Although the conversation around 10,000 hours of purposeful practice creating an expert is nuanced,[12,13] common-sense dictates that the more we practice a skill, the more effective we will be at executing that skill. Surgical simulation allows for the repetitive skills training that improves trainee performance. This allows learners to practice surgical skills in an environment with low stakes so that they are able to execute when they are given an opportunity to do so in the OR. In the orthopedic domain, arthroscopic simulation is more developed and validated than other subspecialty fields in orthopedics,[14,15] and has shown significant benefits to trainees. Simulation lags but is growing in the orthopedic trauma world,[16–18] and there is growing effort to find effective methods that translate fracture reduction and fixation into surgical simulation.

Effective Teaching

There are several steps that can be taken individually to maximize our effectiveness as educators. First and most important, foster an attitude and environment of professionalism. Professionalism serves as a "medical morality," which is a personal quality and an active behavior. It includes honesty, integrity, responsibility, respect for others, compassion, empathy, commitment to self-improvement, and altruism.[19] It includes the promise of help to the vulnerable patient and a commitment to expertise in the field.[20] It is on this foundation that we build the rest of our teaching. If a student does not first respect the quality of your work and the empathy with which you treat patients and students, you will not be maximally effective in your ability to educate them.

Teach them how to learn

A large portion of the information we teach trainees during residency will be outdated by the time they have been in practice for 10 years. Help them identify the way in which they learn best and different sources that best fit their learning style. Reinforce the importance of self-awareness and insight to identify the gaps in their knowledge or skill set. Encourage intentional time set aside at regular intervals, which can be used for planning/goal setting and honest assessment of progress toward achieving previous goals. The regular evaluation of our goals allows for us to develop concrete steps toward achieving them.

Use an active teaching style

Learning is more intense and permanent when the learner is actively engaged.[21,22] We have all sat through 100-slide-long PowerPoint presentations where the attempt at passive knowledge transfer falls flat. We rarely remember more than three slides because we were not engaged and participating with the speaker. Active learning has been shown to be a superior method with educational and psychological studies demonstrating its benefit in early education and in adult learners.[21] Instead of passive learning (eg, reading off a PowerPoint), use the Socratic method and teach through interactive reasoning. In small group sessions, ask challenging (post-graduate-year appropriate), but nonthreatening questions, and allow learners to talk through an answer.[21,22] Questions should relate to key concepts, have a specific purpose, and should demand critical thinking instead of simple regurgitation of facts. In larger group sessions, information should be meaningfully organized, presented clearly, and delivered in manageable chunks, while remaining interactive with the audience. In the OR, make residents read before your case and make it clear what is expected and the consequences if they fall short (if they do not read, they observe and participate only as an assistant).

Although active learning should take place every day, the didactic portion of resident education begins with program planning. It is critical to effective teaching and learning that a clear and well-defined curriculum is used. Each lecture topic should be carefully selected, and have clear objectives. This plan should be subject to evaluation and open to change to evolve and meet the needs of our learners.

Require accountability

Resident performance is driven by the resident's perception of how he or she will be evaluated (residents will figure out how they will be evaluated and seek to excel in this area). Set clear learning objectives and link them to the evaluation.[22] Allow trainees to set specific goals for their time on the rotation. Provide opportunities for learning based on the objectives and individual goals.

Positive peer pressure is used to help foster learning. This does not mean humiliation in front of their peers, because excessive anxiety decreases human ability to process and produces a negative learning environment. However, some stress heightens alertness and improves performance. So, respectfully engage residents based on their level of training, and let them struggle and search for the answer before providing constructive relief. Orthopedic residents are high achievers. When they are aware

of the objectives or an assignment, and know they will be held accountable to that standard, they will be motivated to prepare and/or complete the tasks they have been given. If we do not set the expectation of excellence, we must not be disappointed when it is not achieved.

Give and receive feedback

Accurate and timely feedback is critical for successful teaching. Feedback can range from correcting bad surgical habits and practices to praising empathetic patient interactions. Students learn more if you give feedback that immediately follows the action, thought, or speech that you want to improve or reinforce. Final evaluations encompassing a rotation happen later, but formative feedback happens in real time.[21] This formative evaluation provides actionable information for the purpose of making improvements. When giving feedback, the tried and true method of asking "What went well? What could be done differently? What could be improved on?" is a great place to start. In the summative or final evaluation, address the objectives set out at the beginning of the rotation, and also address the resident's goals.

Feedback is a two-way street. Remember that what is learned is more important than what is taught (they do not always learn what we think we are teaching, make them demonstrate that they understand).[22] We should ask learners if we have effectively taught the objectives. Have a fair and anonymous way that you as a teacher are evaluated by learners. Do not take negative comments personally, but instead look at this feedback as a means to improve your teaching skills. Take the valid points in these evaluations to heart and incorporate this feedback into your teaching style. Look for outside help to grow as a teacher and refine your skills and teaching strategies. The American Academy of Orthopaedic Surgeons and other organizations, such as the like the Arbeitsgemeinschaft für Osteosynthesefragen (AO), have courses dedicated to helping faculty improve their ability to educate. Take advantage of these resources.

Autonomy

In today's practice environment, resident autonomy has been diminished in comparison with a generation ago. Most of the increasing oversight and regulations are designed to increase patient safety, but also resulted in increased fewer surgical repetitions for orthopedic residents and decreased independence of residents in the OR. Despite these challenges, we must still find a way to graduate competent surgeons from our programs.[23] When we do not make concerted efforts to promote (supervised) resident independence and decision making inside and outside the OR, the result is an abrupt transition from assistant to primary decision maker on entering practice.[24] This transition can lead to a crisis of confidence for early practice orthopedic surgeons. Such tools as the Ottawa Surgical Competency Operating Room Evaluation[25] or Zwisch Scale of Progressive Autonomy[26] are used to help quantify the stages of resident autonomy achieved by individual residents. The American Board of Orthopedic Surgeons has begun requiring evaluations of specific core procedures to ensure that we appropriately document surgical competence in trainees.[27] Make a conscious effort to facilitate problem-solving skills, foster leadership skills, and promote independence in those trainees who help us care for patients.

SUMMARY

Healy[28] succinctly sums up the debt we owe to our teachers and the burden we carry as teachers:

> ...please think about your own teachers. Think about what they taught you and think about what you learned from them. Think about how your teachers helped you to accomplish your goals. Think about how you can help your students to accomplish their goals. Teaching and teachers help us to define our lives and our profession. Teachers made a profound difference in my life. As an orthopedic teacher, you can make a difference in the lives of others.

To have a maximally effective career as surgeons and educators, we must seek continual improvement, to be "better today than I was yesterday." This humble pursuit of personal and professional development requires self-awareness of your guiding purpose, your "why," and grit, the passion and perseverance to achieve long-term goals.[3] These thoughts were distilled into a short note from one of my mentors shortly after the fellowship match: "Enjoy and appreciate the chances that you've earned, work really hard, have lots of fun, and be better than just good."

Recognize that educators shape learners by more than what they teach them about orthopedics, and the "hidden curriculum" is equally important as a well-planned didactic curriculum. We teach residents how to obtain a thorough history and physical, and we teach them how to speak to a circulating nurse. We teach them how to perform complex surgical procedures and how to balance work and home life. We teach them how to behave in the clinic, and how to be a good partner. In essence, we teach who we are just as much as what we know. I try remind myself to live every day in a way that proves worthy of that charge. I also remind myself to live humbly, knowing at times I will succeed, and other times I will fail. I know that I will never obtain perfection as a surgeon or as a teacher, but I will forever press on toward that mark.

DISCLOSURE

Clay Spitler is a paid presenter for AO North America, a consultant for Depuy Synthes and KCI, and a salaried employee of Lippincott/Journal of Bone and Joint Surgery.

REFERENCES

1. Gofton W, Regehr G. What we don't know we are teaching: unveiling the hidden curriculum. Clin Orthop Relat Res 2006;449:20–7.
2. London M. The Oxford handbook of lifelong learning. New York: Oxford University Press; 2011.
3. Duckworth A. Grit: the power of passion and perseverance. New York: Scribner; 2016.
4. Saint Augustine of Hippo, 354-430. The Confessions of Saint Augustine. Mount Vernon: White Plains, NY: Peter Pauper Press, 19401949.
5. Warren R. The purpose-driven life: what on earth am I here for? Grand Rapids (MI): Zondervan; 2002.
6. Ou AY, Waldman DA, Peterson SJ. Do humble CEOs matter? An examination of CEO humility and firm outcomes. J Manag 2018;44(3):1147–73.
7. Bryant K. The Mamba mentality: how I play. New York: MCD, Farrar, Straus and Girou; 2018.
8. Willink J, Babin L. Extreme ownership: how U.S. Navy SEALs lead and win. 2nd edition. New York: St. Martin's Press; 2017.
9. Kelly JD 4th. Your best life: valuing emotional intelligence-lessons from the Super Bowl champions. Clin Orthop Relat Res 2018;476(12):2328–30.
10. Institute for Health and Human Potential. What is emotional intelligence?. Available at: https://www.ihhp.com/meaning-ofemotional-intelligence. Accessed August 21, 2020.
11. Ovans A. How emotional intelligence became a key leadership skill. Available at: https://hbr.org/2015/04/how-emotionalintelligence-became-a-key-leadership-skill. Accessed August 20, 2020.
12. Gladwell M. Outliers: the story of success. New York: Little, Brown and Company; 2008.

13. Ericsson A, Pool R. Peak: secrets from the new science of expertise. Boston, MA: Houghton Mifflin Harcourt; 2016.

14. Bartlett JD, Lawrence JE, Stewart ME, et al. Does virtual reality simulation have a role in training trauma and orthopaedic surgeons? Bone Joint J 2018;100-B(5):559–65.

15. Rashed S, Ahrens PM, Maruthainar N, et al. The role of arthroscopic simulation in teaching surgical skills: a systematic review of the literature. JBJS Rev 2018;6(9):e8.

16. Christian MW, Griffith C, Schoonover C, et al. Construct validation of a novel hip fracture fixation surgical simulator. J Am Acad Orthop Surg 2018; 26(19):689–97.

17. Weber A, Domes C, Christian M, et al. Effect of training modules on hip fracture surgical skills simulation performance: early validation of the AAOS/OTA simulator. J Bone Joint Surg Am 2019;101(22):2051–60.

18. Yehyawi TM, Thomas TP, Ohrt GT, et al. A simulation trainer for complex articular fracture surgery. J Bone Joint Surg Am 2013;95(13):e92.

19. Zuckerman JD, Holder JP, Mercuri JJ, et al. Teaching professionalism in orthopaedic surgery residency programs. J Bone Joint Surg Am 2012;94(8):e51.

20. Pellegrino ED. Toward a reconstruction of medical morality. Am J Bioeth 2006;6(2):65–71.

21. Ahn J, Achor TS. Tips for being an effective teacher. J Orthop Trauma 2014;28(Suppl 9): S15–7.

22. Pinney SJ, Mehta S, Pratt DD, et al. Orthopaedic surgeons as educators. Applying the principles of adult education to teaching orthopaedic residents. J Bone Joint Surg Am 2007;89(6):1385–92.

23. Dougherty PJ, Cannada LK, Murray P, et al. Progressive autonomy in the era of increased supervision: AOA critical issues. J Bone Joint Surg Am 2018;100(18):e122.

24. LaPorte DM, Tornetta P, Marsh JL. Challenges to orthopaedic resident education. J Am Acad Orthop Surg 2019;27(12):419–25.

25. Gofton WT, Dudek NL, Wood TJ, et al. The Ottawa Surgical Competency Operating Room Evaluation (O-SCORE): a tool to assess surgical competence. Acad Med 2012;87(10):1401–7.

26. DaRosa DA, Zwischenberger JB, Meyerson SL, et al. A theory-based model for teaching and assessing residents in the operating room. J Surg Educ 2013; 70:24–30.

27. ABOS/CORD Surgical Skill Assessment Program. Available at: https://www.abos.org/wp-content/uploads/2019/02/abos_cord_surgical_skills_assessment_program.pdf. Accessed August 22, 2020.

28. Healy WL. Thoughts on teaching (for orthopaedic graduates). J Bone Joint Surg Am 2011;93(1):e1.

The Role of Mentoring in the Professional Identity Formation of Medical Students

Kristen A. Bettin, MD, MEd[a,b,*]

KEYWORDS

• Professional identity formation • Mentoring • Medical students • Orthopedics

---

KEY POINTS

- Professional identity formation is a lifelong, iterative process whereby a medical student develops a sense of self and embodies the ideals and values of a physician.
- Socialization is key for the formation of professional identity for medical students, including formal and informal curriculum, clinical experiences, role modeling, and mentorship and narrative reflection.
- Of these, positive mentoring relationships with experienced faculty members has been shown to improve students' satisfaction with their career choices, boost confidence in career choices, and give them an opportunity to form their professional identity in a safe, nurturing environment.
- For orthopedics, successful mentoring can encourage medical students to choose a career in orthopedic surgery and supports students in their development of their own identity as future surgeons.
- Positive orthopedic faculty mentors also may improve matriculation of underrepresented minorities and women into the field and profession of orthopedic surgery.

INTRODUCTION

In the 1990s and early 2000s, there was a big emphasis on teaching professionalism in undergraduate medical education, with a focus on how to act and behave as a physician. More recently, however, the focus has shifted from teaching professionalism to expanding to the concept of professional identity formation (PIF) for medical students. Although the formal and informal (hidden) curricula of medical school are important tools for teaching medical students about professionalism and professional identity, there are other means with which to teach medical students about this lifelong process of PIF. These tools include narrative reflection and socialization, in addition to formal teaching.[1] Clinical experiences, role modeling, and mentoring all play pivotal roles in the socialization process of third-year medical students with regard to their PIF. This review specifically defines PIF for medical students, discussing factors that influence PIF, exploring the role of mentoring on the PIF of medical students, and suggesting ways to use mentoring and PIF to increase interest of medical students, especially women and underrepresented minority students, in the field of orthopedics.

PROFESSIONALISM VERSUS PROFESSIONAL IDENTITY FORMATION

Professionalism incorporates the expected attitudes and behaviors of members of a given profession, in this case medicine.[2] Medical professionalism often incorporates ideas, such

---

[a] Department of Pediatrics, University of Tennessee Health Science Center College of Medicine, 49 North Dunlap Street, FOB 149, Memphis, TN 38103, USA; [b] Department of Medical Education, University of Tennessee Health Science Center College of Medicine, 49 North Dunlap Street, FOB 149, Memphis, TN 38103, USA
* Corresponding author.
E-mail address: kbettin@uthsc.edu

Orthop Clin N Am 52 (2021) 61–68
https://doi.org/10.1016/j.ocl.2020.08.007

as ethical treatment of patients, self-awareness, accountability, respect for patients, teamwork, and social responsibility.[2] Professionalism has been identified as a core clinical competency for medical residents by the Accreditation Council for Graduate Medical Education, which has been extrapolated nearly universally to undergraduate medical education evaluation and assessment tools.[3] Medical students learn this sense of "right and wrong" through explicit didactic teaching but also through direct observation of the behaviors and actions of role models in the clinical and academic setting. Professionalism lends itself toward a dichotomy of right/wrong, good/bad, or acceptable/unacceptable.

Some authors have described a period of "proto-professionalism" for medical students, emphasizing this time in medical school where learners are educated on the domains of professionalism and work to attain professionalism as they move throughout their medical training.[4] Although the tenets of professionalism are clearer, achieving professionalism is a process that takes years to attain and a lifetime to maintain.[4]

PIF, by contrast, is more complex and nuanced. It is a lifelong, iterative, and continuous process of incorporating the beliefs, values, and morals of the profession of medicine into one's sense of self.[5] Professional identity is the combination of one's personal identity with that of the desired profession to yield a cohesive identity that incorporates elements of clinical practice, expertise, professional attitudes and behaviors, and self-actualization in medicine. Cruess and colleagues[6(p1447)] more eloquently described a physician's professional identity as "a representation of self, achieved in stages over time during which the characteristics, values, and norms of the medical profession are internalized, resulting in an individual thinking, acting, and feeling like a physician." Many authors have suggested that PIF occurs through a series of steps, whereas some liken it to a more continuous process of construct identity destruction and recreation.[6,7] Still others discuss the idea of students reaching a "common identity" or becoming one of the group (of physicians) prior to reaching their own individualized professional identity.[8] This type of herd mentality is important for students' identity formation because they generally begin this journey of becoming a physician as feeling like an outsider. The confidence they gain from being part of the medical team propels them forward into their own professional identity. Given the importance of the development of professional identity on a medical student's sense of self, more recently some medical educators have advocated for the integration of identity formation into medical education curricula much in the way the core competencies have been integrated.[6,7]

PROCESS OF IDENTITY FORMATION

As part of the formal teaching of professionalism and PIF, clinicians can and should engage students in experiential learning and role-modeling.[2] Many investigators also have described various learning theories as they relate to the formation of professional identity for medical students. Goldie[9] explains the concept of "multiple identities" whereby the student's professional identity is formed by the interplay between the student's ego identity, personal, identity, and social identity, which are influenced by personality, interaction (with role models, patients, and so forth) and social structure (ie, being a member of the medical team and observing the hidden curriculum of medical school.) Social identity theory similarly focuses on the student's ability to conform with the in-group and assimilate into the group with which they hope to identify.[9]

Frost and Regehr[10] suggest a social constructionist theory of identity formation that is based on the discourses (opposing social constructs) of standardization and diversity in medical education. In this view, students are exposed to the competing ideals of standardization (a set of expected behaviors, attitudes, and characteristics required of physicians; meeting the "norms") and diversity (the components of the personal identity that make a student stand out including gender, race, sexual orientation, religion, ethnicity, and socioeconomic status prior to medical school). These competing forces cause students to construct a professional identity and navigate the cognitive dissonance they may feel between 2 opposing sets of values.

These theories come up short, however, when discussing the holistic process of PIF. Professional identity is not just belonging to the in-group but rather how the student internalizes the beliefs and values of the in-group and incorporates them into his/her own sense of professional self. Jarvis-Selinger and colleagues[7(p1185,1186)] nicely melded these ideas of multiple identities by describing identity formation as "an adaptive developmental process that happens simultaneously at 2 levels: (1) at the level of the individual, which involves the psychological development of the person and (2) at the collective level, which involves the socialization of the person into appropriate roles and forms of participation in the community's work," with the community being that of the medical community.

FACTORS INFLUENCING PIF

Many factors affect the formation of professional identity of medical students. Studies state that a combination of prior experiences; formal and informal (hidden) curriculum; socialization— including clinical encounters, role models, and mentors; and narrative reflection aid in the formation of professional identity.[5,6] The informal or hidden curriculum of medical school — the dissonance between what is taught to students in a professional sense and what is observed by students regarding behaviors and interactions of attending physicians or residents — may also be a major influencer of professional identity.[9]

More recently, however, socialization has been touted as the main tenet of PIF and incorporates clinical encounters and role models and the conscious and unconscious observations of students in these areas, including self-reflection.[1,7] Common socializing agents in the clinical encounters include physicians, other health care professionals, and even the student's own peer group.[7] Emphasis has been placed on the role of prior experiences and personal identities and their interactions with students' personal narrative reflections about clinical experiences as a means for PIF.[5,6] Wong and Trollope-Kumar[5] were able to qualitatively demonstrate a progression in PIF for medical students engaging in narrative reflections throughout their preclinical curriculum. Themes that evolved from these narratives included prior experiences, role models, patient encounters, curriculum, and societal expectations. Throughout the course of these preclinical exercises, students were able to reflect on their initial feelings of being overwhelmed and with inadequate knowledge base and clinical skills to manage patients. Through their experiences with witnessed patient encounters and interactions with mentors, they were able to shape their awareness of the nuanced aspects of professional identity in medicine and their role in this profession.

The investigators noted that both positive and negative mentors can have an impact on PIF in either a positive or negative way, depending on the circumstances of the encounter.[5] Regardless of which theory is ascribed to with regard to the PIF of medical students, nearly every theory expounds on the importance of role models and mentors in the process of identity formation.[1,2,5,7–9] However, mentors should be mindful of the power differentials and presence of potential biases in mentoring relationships that may affect students' identity formation.[9] Thus, the role of medical professionals and clinician educators is to find and become effective mentors for students who will provide them with the safe space to explore their professional identities.

ROLE MODELING IN MEDICINE

Cruess and colleagues[1] outline the role of socialization in the development of professional identity for medical students. One of the most profound components of socialization is interactions with role models. Many studies suggest that role modeling (both positive and negative) has an impact on students' development of their professional identity.[1,5] The most significant interactions of students with role models are no doubt in the clinical rotations. Students are able to observe attending physicians and residents in action and learn from not only what they say but also what these experienced physicians do and how they act.

Interactions of students and junior physicians with senior or experienced physicians during teaching sessions (ie, morning report) also can provide powerful modeling of clinical acumen, critical thinking, and disease management but may be lacking on the softer side of medicine, such as humanism.[8] Although these educational interactions no doubt are beneficial, more individualized role modeling may have an even bigger impact on students' sense of self as physicians.

Although role-modeling alone is not sufficient for the formation of professional identity,[1,5,8] it can be incorporated into other forms of socialization to enhance students PIF. Role models, either through discussion about clinical experiences or through feedback from personal reflective narratives, can help guide students to work through difficult experiences, turning these potentially detrimental or sentinel events into opportunities for learning and growth.[5] Although positive role modeling itself promotes PIF, so can discussion and reflection of negative experiences. Having invested role models and mentors that provide a safe area for students to discuss their negative experiences can help shape those experiences into profound learning opportunities and a more positively directed professional identity rather than increasing cynicism and discontent. Role models can serve as moderators for students' self-reflections about negative clinical or educational experiences to put into perspective their own goals and aspirations for their professional identity. Frost and Regehr[10] support that students should seek mentors to discuss professional identity and the discourse that they encounter in the clinical settings. This is important especially for combating the "hidden" curriculum in medical school, meaning the dissonance between what is expected of physicians and what is observed by students with regard to mistreatment, disrespect, discrimination, bias, and any other multitude of similar negative experiences.[5]

ROLE MODELING AND MENTORING

Role modeling and mentoring sometimes are used interchangeably in medical education and although an experienced clinician can serve in both roles, they are indeed different. Whereas role modeling is viewed more as a pedagogical approach to PIF with passive observation by the medical student,[8] mentoring is more than this. Mentorship is an active ongoing process that requires preparation, dedication, and investment of time from both the mentor and the mentee. Mentoring is "a relationship, formal and/or informal, between a novice and one more senior persons in the field for the purposes of career and personal development and preparation for leadership."[11(p1089)]

Effective mentor-mentee relationships are key to the success of mentorship.[12,13] Thus, faculty must gain rapport with and show mutual respect for students in order to provide meaningful mentorship. Outlining clear expectations and identifying goals with the student on the front end also are important for effective mentoring.[12,13]

Other characteristics that are crucial for successful mentoring relationships are trust, accountability, mutual respect, reciprocity, personal connection, and shared interests and values between the mentor and mentee.[12,13] Not surprisingly, mentoring relationships are more successful when mentees are able to choose a mentor with similar career or specialty interests and when the mentoring relationship is initiated by the mentee.[12-14] The ability to have open discussions and maintain transparency, while also protecting confidentiality, also were cited as important aspects of a successful mentoring relationship for mentees.[12]

Through a qualitative study, Straus and colleagues[13] were able to identify additional characteristics of effective mentors, which included altruism, honesty, trustworthiness, accessibility, the ability of the mentor to be an active listener, mentorship experience, and professional experience. Mentoring, however, is a 2-way street. Educators, also must teach mentees to embody the characteristics of effective mentees, including active listening and openness to feedback, taking responsibility and initiative for the mentoring relationship, preparing for mentoring meetings and being respectful of stated timelines.[13]

In contrast, overdependence on the mentor for guidance, poor communication, conflicts of interest (eg, mentor being an evaluator or supervisor of the mentee or competition between mentor and mentee), paternalistic mentors, time constraints or lack of commitment to mentoring, poor mentoring skills or lack of mentoring experience (focusing on the mentors ideas rather than developing the mentee's), lack of institutional support (financially or in the form of protected academic time), personality differences, and unrealistic expectations all tend to erode mentoring relationships.[11-13] Pellegrini[15] succinctly sums up these ideas as 4 key principles of surgical mentoring: style, ego, selection, and time.

The optimal frequency of mentoring interactions is not explicitly reported; however, regular communication, anywhere from a monthly to semiannually, depending on the needs of the student/mentee, is key to successful mentoring.[11,12] Factors that may affect frequency and goals of mentoring include personal characteristics, age, specialty, type of practice, gender, and career goals.[11]

Successful mentorship also encompasses factors outside of the individuals, mentor and mentee, involved in the mentoring relationship. Wilson[11] described several systemic barriers to effective mentoring, in addition to some of the personal barriers, discussed previously, which include (1) the authoritative culture of medicine, in particular surgical fields, that does not value seeking help; (2) lack of time; (3) the fact that no one mentor can provide all mentoring needs to a specific mentee (ie, need for multiple mentors per mentee); and (4) lack of institutional support. Institutions must support the time and effort of faculty mentors, and mentees also must be afforded the ability to select a different mentor without retaliation or recrimination if the mentoring relationship is not mutually beneficial.[11]

Faculty development is key for success which may include workshops on mentoring, the use of checklists to guide mentoring discussion, and feedback from mentees,[6,13] as are resources to support such services, such as protected time for faculty and institutional support of mentorship programs.[11,15]

DISCUSSION
Mentoring as a Means of Professional Identity Formation for Medical Students

Frost and Regehr describe medical educators as the "gatekeepers" for "producing the right kind of physician."[10(p1570)] With this charge, clinicians and medical educators are tasked with the goal of mentoring medical students into successful physicians. Career advising, advocacy on the student's behalf (eg, for a residency interview), networking (via national conferences or organizations), creating opportunities (eg, research and article writing), goal setting, and career monitoring all are important aspects of the mentoring role for medical students,[13] and, in fact, many mentors view their role as just that, an academic or career advisor. The role of mentor, however, especially in the context of PIF, goes beyond the career advising of how many residency programs to which students should apply, how many and from whom they should obtain letters of recommendation, or to which program(s) to seek away rotations. Mentorship extends to the process of supporting the student through his/her journey to think, act, and do as a physician.

"Good mentors [are] able to identify potential strengths and limitations in their mentees and promote their career development."[13] This process of providing formative feedback and constructive criticism is an important part of PIF and can be utilized within the safe environment of the mentor-mentee relationship in order to further contribute to the PIF of the mentee.

In addition to career guidance and advising, offering emotional support and exploring work/life balance also are critical to the mentor's role.[13] Mentors also provide a safe and welcoming environment for honest and transparent reflection on life events, clinical experiences, and mentees' goals and aspirations.[8,12]

This role of providing emotional support, of being a nurturer, often is counterintuitive to the previously discussed construct of a surgeon's professional identity. Pellegrini[15] highlighted this conflict nicely in his 2009 presidential address to the American Orthopaedic Association, stating, "An effective mentor is the guardian and promoter of the young physicians' personal and professional development. So, mentoring is the act of nurturing the emotional and intellectual growth of another person to

the point that, and here comes the hard part, he or she is your peer and equal and, ideally, has eclipsed your own accomplishments with the tools and opportunities that you have provided." Most do not presume that a fourth-year medical student whom they have mentored is their equal in a professional sense as in the way a fifth-year orthopedic resident or junior faculty member may become. Yet, Pellegrini's address touches on other key success measures in mentoring: the mentor must transcend his or her own successes to promote and derive satisfaction from the successes of the mentee, while recognizing that successful mentoring relationships are mutually beneficial with regard to personal and professional development of both mentor and mentee.[15,16]

Mentoring of Prospective Orthopedic Trainees

Several studies have shown that early exposure to musculoskeletal and orthopedic coursework and exposure to orthopedic mentors can increase students' interest in orthopedic surgery.[17,18] Both medical students and residents believe that mentorship is helpful and important for career development, and a majority of surveyed residents in 1 study felt that mentorship should be part of residency training.[14] Self-selected mentors typically result in more satisfying mentoring relationships from the prospective of the mentee[12–14]; thus, it may be prudent to allow trainees to choose their own mentors. In 1 study of orthopedic surgery residents, mentees who self-selected their mentor found mentors to be more helpful aiding in career decisions and professional development, supporting their education, and in providing opportunities for networking.[14] These residents noted approachability, subspecialty interest, similar research interests, reputation as a mentor, and ideal practice environment as desirable characteristics of mentors.[14] In the conclusion of this study, the investigators suggest that mentoring programs should be developed in every orthopedic residency program and that residents should be encouraged to seek mentors early in their postgraduate training in order to cultivate these relationships throughout residency.[14] To them, I say, why wait?

In a 2017 survey of medical students from 10 institutions, the factors that influenced them the most in selecting their career specialty were specialty content and quality of life/lifestyle/stress level.[17] For students considering orthopedics as a career, however, compared with students who were not interested in orthopedics, the factors of experience as a patient, anticipated income, and prestige of a specialty were significantly more influential than factors, such as length of training, quality of life/lifestyle/stress level within a specialty, and gender diversity within the speciality.[17] A mentor in the field of orthopedic surgery is primely situated to provide both information about the specialty content and also other factors of life and career that could potentially influence medical students' decision to pursue orthopedics.

Using Mentoring and Professional Identify Formation to Increase Diversity in Orthopedics

Orthopedics is, unfortunately, known as one of the least diverse medical specialties. As of the Association of American Medical Colleges (AAMC) data from 2019 to 2020, although women now make up 52% of matriculants to US medical schools,[19] only approximately 15% of active orthopedic residents in the United States are women, the lowest percentage of any of residency training program for post-graduate year 1 (PGY-1) residents.[20] There are multiple postulated reasons for this large discrepancy of women in orthopedics, but it is clear that there is concern for this imbalance in orthopedics. Referring back to the survey by Rao and colleagues,[17] among men and women students interested in orthopedics, women were more influenced by gender and racial diversity and less influenced by income and prestige of the specialty, compared with men.

In order to increase diversity in a field where little exists, practicing surgeons should utilize mentorship. Medical students report positive influence of mentors on their career specialty decision.[17,18] Race/ethnicity of the mentor compared with the mentee does not seem to be as influential, but sex of the mentor is.[17] Both men and women students report that same-sex mentors have a stronger influence on career specialty choice than opposite-sex mentors.[17] This presents an obvious problem for attracting women students to the field of orthopedics: there are few practicing female orthopedic surgeons. Orthopedic surgery departments should consider focused efforts on recruiting women orthopedic surgeons to help produce a pipeline of mentoring for women medical students.[17,18,21]

Many medical students applying to orthopedics may feel the competing discourses of standardization and diversity discussed by Frost and Regehr.[10] Women and underrepresented minority students may either feel disadvantaged because they do not fit the standard stereotype of an orthopedic surgery residency applicant, or they may feel at an advantage because the same characteristics that cause them to deviate from the stereotype also help them to stand out.

Lack of interest in specialty content seems to be the primary reason for decreased interest in orthopedics for women and minority students according to Rao and colleagues,[17] which may be related either to lack of exposure to musculoskeletal content early on in medical school (although this was a decidedly less influencing factor), lack of mentors, both, or neither. O'Connor,[18] however, found evidence of perceived or actual gender bias to be a potential concern for fewer women in the field of orthopedics.[18] In her review, lack of access to women orthopedic mentors, perceptions of how women fit into the specialty of orthopedics, and gender bias in the form of illegal residency interview questions regarding marital status, family planning, gender, and children all may contribute negatively to women's perspectives of orthopedics as career.[18] Positive influencing factors for women interested in orthopedics were exposure to orthopedics and musculoskeletal disease early in medical school, and, not surprisingly, mentors in the field. Thus, residency programs, departments of orthopedics, and medical schools should consider early introduction of orthopedics into the medical school curriculum while fostering longitudinal mentoring relationships in orthopedics.[17,18,21]

Although orthopedic departments across the country should continue to recruit women orthopedic surgeons to mentor medical students, there still are not enough same-sex mentors for all potentially interested women medical students. Thus, as a specialty, efforts should be made to improve the mentoring skills for all surgeons, regardless of gender or racial/ethnical background in order to improve mentoring opportunities for all students interested in orthopedics, especially women and minority students. Medical schools and residency programs also can actively engage in improving mentorship capabilities through mentorship programs with residents and faculty.

Students interested in orthopedics can take advantage of several mentoring and pipeline programs and resources, many of these specifically focused on women and minority medical students, including: Perry Initiative Medical Student Outreach Program[22,23] (for women medical students), Nth Dimensions,[24,25] Ruth Jackson Orthopaedic Society,[26] J. Robert Gladden Orthopaedic Society,[25,27] American Association of Latino Orthopaedic Surgeons,[28] American

Academy of Orthopaedic Surgeons (AAOS) Diversity Advisory Board,[29] New York University Summer Externship Program[30] (for underrepresented minorities), Duke University Feagin Leadership Program,[31] Ruth Jackson Orthopaedic Society *Guide for Women in Orthopedic Surgery*[32] (a guidebook for women in orthopedics), AAOS medical student program at the AAOS annual meeting.[29] Two of these programs have demonstrated positive impact on the tendency for women and underrepresented minority student participants to have increased rate of applying to or matching into orthopedics residencies.[22,24]

SUMMARY

Physician educators and mentors can offer personal guidance, academic support, and the ability for students to reflect on the components of their personal identity and how this personal identity informs and contributes to their professional identity. As others have alluded to, surgeons, including orthopedic surgeons, may not be natural-born mentors[11,15,21,33]; cultivation of effective mentors and mentorship skills is necessary for successful mentoring of surgical trainees. Thus, coming back to the idea that for mentorship to be truly successful in terms of mentee PIF, the mentors must be willing to set aside their own aspirations and mentor future generations of physicians and surgeons for the greater good of the medical community and future patients. This is true of mentoring relationships with medical students. Many clinician educators have thought at some point in their late (or early) career, I would never have gotten into medical school, residency, this job, etc., nowadays compared with these applicants.

As the competitiveness for medical school and residency positions continues to skyrocket, especially for residencies, such as orthopedics, mentors in the field have the distinct position to help guide students to their realities and callings. And, a calling it often is.[15] The ability to learn to "[revel] in succession planning and [derive] personal pleasure from the accomplishments of those arounds us requires a realization we are each mortal and capable of only a finite contribution to this existence."[15] Mentorship is a way continue the ideals, values, skills, culture, research, and innovation in a specialty and helps ensure that a new generation of diverse trainees understands the gravity and embodies the depth of what it means to be an orthopedic surgeon.

CLINICS CARE POINTS

- Mentoring, as part of socialization, has a positive impact on students' PIF and career specialty choice.
- Characteristics of effective mentoring relationships include mutual respect, clear expectations and goal setting, accountability, reciprocity, personal connection, shared interests and values between the mentor and mentee, and self-selected mentors.
- Characteristics of effective mentors include altruism, honesty, trustworthiness, accessibility, active listening, mentorship experience, and professional experience.
- Failed mentoring relationships often are due to overdependence on the mentor for guidance, poor communication, conflicts of interest, paternalistic mentors, time constraints, poor mentoring, lack of institutional support, personality differences, and/or unrealistic expectations.
- Medical students who have an orthopedic surgeon mentor and have early exposure to orthopedics in medical school are more likely to consider a career in orthopedics.
- Effective mentoring and pipeline programs can increase the chance of women and underrepresented minority medical students to pursue a career in orthopedics.

DISCLOSURE

The author has nothing to disclose.

REFERENCES

1. Cruess RL, Cruess SR, Boudreau JD, et al. A schematic representation of the professional identity formation and socialization of medical students and residents: a guide for medical educators. Acad Med 2015;90:718–25.
2. Cruess RL. Teaching professionalism: theory, principles, practices. Clin Orthop Relat Res 2006;449:177–85.
3. Holmboe ES, Edgar L, Hamstra S. Accreditation council on graduate medical education the milestones guidebook. 2016. Available at: https://www.acgme.org/Portals/0/MilestonesGuidebook.pdf (finish citation). Accessed April 28, 2020.
4. Hilton SR, Slotnick HB. Proto-professionalism: how professionalization occurs across the continuum of medical education. Med Educ 2005;39:58–65.

5. Wong A, Trollope-Kumar K. Reflections: an inquiry into medical students' professional identity formation. Med Educ 2014;48:489–501.

6. Cruess RL, Cruess SR, Boudreau JD, et al. Reframing medical education to support professional identity formation. Acad Med 2014;89(11):1446–51.

7. Jarvis-Selinger S, Pratt DD, Regehr G. Competency is not enough: integrating identity formation into the medical education discourse. Acad Med 2012; 87:1185–90.

8. Wilson I, Cowin LS, Johnson M, et al. Professional identity in medical students: pedagogical challenges to medical education. Teach Learn Med 2013;25(4):369–73.

9. Goldie J. The formation of professional identity in medical students: Considerations for educators. Med Teach 2012;34:e641–8.

10. Frost HD, Regehr G. "I AM a doctor": negotiating the discourses of standardization and diversity in professional identity construction. Acad Med 2013;88(10):1570–7.

11. Wilson FC. Mentoring in orthopaedics: an evolving need for nuture. J Bone Joint Surg Am 2004;86-A(5):1089–91.

12. Sng JH, Pei Y, Toh YP, et al. Mentoring relationships between senior physicians and junior doctors and/or medical students: a thematic review. Med Teach 2017;39(8):866–75.

13. Straus SE, Johnson MO, Marquez C, et al. Characteristics of successful and failed mentoring relationships: a qualitative study across two academic health centers. Acad Med 2013;88:82–9.

14. Flint JH, Jahangir A, Browner BD, et al. The value of mentorship in orthopaedic surgery resident education: the residents' perspective. J Bone Joint Surg Am 2009;91:1017–22.

15. Pellegrini VD. Mentoring: our obligation...our heritage. J Bone Joint Surg Am 2009;91:2511–9.

16. Pellegrini VD. Mentoring during residency education: a unique challenge for the surgeon? Clin Orthop Relat Res 2006;449:143–8.

17. Rao RD, Khatib ON, Agarwal A. Factors motivating medical students in selecting a career specialty: relevance for a robust orthopaedic pipeline. J Am Acad Orthop Surg 2017;25:527–35.

18. O'Connor MI. Medical school experiences shape women students' interests in orthopaedic surgery. Clin Orthop Relat Res 2016;474:1967–72.

19. Association of American Medical Colleges: Matriculants to U.S. medical schools by selected combinations of race/ethnicity and sex, 2016-2017 through 2019-2020. 2019. Available at: https://www.aamc.org/system/files/2019-11/2019_FACTS_Table_A-8.pdf. Accessed May 1, 2020.

20. Association of American Medical Colleges: Report on Residents Table B3. Number of Active Residents, by Type of Medical School, GME Specialty, Sex. 2019. Available at: https://www.aamc.org/data-reports/students-residents/interactive-data/report-residents/2019/table-b3-number-active-residents-type-medical-school-gme-specialty-and-sex. Accessed May 1, 2020.

21. Mulcahey MK, Waterman BR, Hart R, et al. The role of mentoring in the development of successful orthopaedic surgeons. J Am Acad Orthop Surg 2018;26:463–71.

22. Lattanza LL, Meszaros-Dearolf L, O'Connor MI, et al. The Perry Initiative's Medical Student Outreach Program recruits women into orthopaedic residency. Clin Orthop Relat Res 2016;474: 1962–6.

23. The Perry Initiative. Outreach Program. 2020. Available at: https://perryinitiative.org/outreach-programs/. Accessed May 1, 2020.

24. Mason BS, Ross W, Ortega G, et al. Can a strategic pipeline initiative increase the number of women and underrepresented minorities in orthopaedic surgery? Clin Orthop Relat Res 2016;474: 1979–85.

25. Nth Dimesions. Medical Students. Available at: http://www.nthdimensions.org/medical-students. Accessed May 1, 2020.

26. Ruth Jackson Orthopaedic Society. Available at: http://www.rjos.org/. Accessed May 1, 2020.

27. J. Robert Gladden Orthopaedic Society. 2020. Available at: http://www.gladdensociety.org/. Accessed May 1, 2020.

28. American Association of Latino Orthopaedic Surgeons. Available at: https://www.aalos.org/. Accessed May 1, 2020.

29. American Association of Orthopaedic Surgeons Medical Student Program. Available at: https://aaos.org/membership/member-resources/career-development/medical-student-resources/. Accessed May 1, 2020.

30. NYU Orthopaedic Surgery Summer Externship Program. Available at: https://med.nyu.edu/departments-institutes/orthopedic-surgery/education/medical-student-education/summer-externship-program. Accessed May 1, 2020.

31. Duke University: Feagin Leadership Program. Available at: https://www.feaginleadership.org/. Accessed May 1, 2020.

32. Ruth Jackson Orthopaedic Society. RJOS Guide for Women in Orthopaedic Surgery. Available at: http://www.rjos.org/. Accessed May 1, 2020.

33. Cope A, Bezemer J, Mavroveli S, et al. What attitudes and values are incorporated into self as part of professional identity construction when becoming a surgeon? Acad Med 2017;92:544–9.

The Current State of the Residency Match

Jennings H. Dooley, BS[a], Kristen A. Bettin, MD, MEd[b,*], Clayton C. Bettin, MD[c]

KEYWORDS

• Match • Orthopedics • Orthopedics match • NRMP

KEY POINTS

- Each year, the orthopedic surgery residency application pool consists of hundreds of highly competitive applicants that residency programs must be able to efficiently and effectively sort through.
- Identifying well-qualified candidates with the aptitude to become competent, caring surgeons is critical to the continued success and growth of orthopedic surgery.
- In an increasingly diverse world, it is critical that representation within orthopedic surgery better reflects that of the general population to provide the best possible care to patients.

INTRODUCTION

Every year, fourth-year medical students across the country prepare for the most important day of their preceding education: Match Day. It is the culmination of 4 years of medical school; the day when each graduating student learns where they will spend the next few years of their life training to be an independent physician. Students who are "matched" with a residency program have a sure path after graduating medical school to continue their training and become attending physicians on completion of residency. For students who are not "matched" with a residency program, they must find an alternate plan, such as entering the Supplemental Offer Acceptance Program with the hopes of finding an unfilled residency position in their specialty of interest or a surgical/medical preliminary year, or taking a research year with the hopes of reapplying to the Match the next year. In a study of unmatched orthopedic applicants from 1994 to 2013, 56 out of 141 (40%) reapplicants matched into orthopedic surgery the following year. Of those who matched,

37.5% matched at their home institution and 87.5% matched at a program in the same region where they had completed either medical school or a postgraduate year, highlighting the importance of developing meaningful relationships with faculty to successfully match as a reapplicant.[1]

In 2018%, 92% of US allopathic seniors matched to their preferred specialty. However, in orthopedic surgery the match rate is much lower with only 82% of US allopathic senior applicants matching into orthopedics in 2019. This is third lowest specialty match rate behind interventional radiology at 58% and dermatology at 82%, making orthopedic surgery one of the most increasingly competitive fields in medicine.[2]

The purpose of the Match is multifaceted. From the applicant perspective, matching is necessary to continue one's medical training and to become a practicing physician. From the program perspective, the purpose of the Match is to fill residency positions and maintain the pipeline for developing and training future

[a] University of Tennessee Health Science Center College of Medicine, 1190 Isle View Drive, Memphis, TN 38103, USA; [b] University of Tennessee Health Science Center College of Medicine, Departments of Pediatrics and Medical Education, 49 North Dunlap Street, FOB 149, Memphis, TN 38103, USA; [c] Orthopaedic Foot & Ankle Surgery, Department of Orthopaedic Surgery & Biomedical Engineering, University of Tennessee-Campbell Clinic, 1211 Union Avenue, Ste 500, Memphis, TN 38104, USA
* Corresponding author.
E-mail address: kbettin@uthsc.edu

Orthop Clin N Am 52 (2021) 69–76
https://doi.org/10.1016/j.ocl.2020.08.006

physicians. Beyond fulfilling these basic needs, an additional goal of the Match is to ensure that the applicant is a good fit for the residency program in which they are placed. This concept originated in 1952 in response to increasing pressure of medical students to accept internships as early as the beginning of M3 year without yet knowing about potential future offers. It was updated to an "applicant-proposing" algorithm in 1998, which places an applicant into a residency position based on the applicant's rank order list.[3]

Leading up to the Match, there are multiple phases of the application cycle. The first phase takes place from the time an applicant submits their application to the Electronic Residency Application Service (ERAS) to the time they receive invitations for interviews. The second phase takes place from the interview dates to rank order lists due date. For orthopedic surgery, the first phase is largely dominated by objective criteria, such as US Medical Licensing Examination (USMLE) Step 1 score, Alpha Omega Alpha Honor Medical Society (AOA) status, and third-year clerkship grades, which residency program directors use to screen applicants. The second phase allows room for subjective criteria, such as applicant performance during the interview and interactions with faculty, residents, and staff at a given program.[4]

This paper assesses the current state of the orthopedic surgery residency match, analyzing the utility of current applicant screening methods in producing future generations of competent surgeons. It also acknowledges upcoming changes to the residency application process, including the anticipated change of the USMLE Step 1 examination becoming pass/fail, and the unanticipated changes as a result of the current COVID-19 pandemic. Although the current orthopedic residency application process has successfully filled 99% of PGY-1 positions for the 2019 and 2020 application cycles, the process can be improved. Potential improvements to the residency match process include identifying and using predictive factors of resident success in the applicant screening process, finding better ways to match applicants with programs where they will be a good fit, and increasing female and underrepresented minorities within orthopedics.

APPLICANT SCREENING

Each year, the orthopedic surgery residency application pool consists of hundreds of highly competitive applicants that residency programs must be able to efficiently and effectively sort through. With an average of 83 applications per candidate, program directors are faced with an average of 124 applications per resident position and must rely heavily on objective factors and standardization to manage the volume of applications.[5] According to a 2016 survey of program directors from 113 orthopedic surgery residency programs, USMLE Step 1 is the most common screening criteria used by residency programs with 83% of programs having a minimum Step 1 score requirement to be considered for an interview. Fifty-three percent of programs require a minimum score of 230, and 21% require a minimum of 240. Programs directors often cite high volume of applications as the primary driver for having a Step 1 cutoff score.[6] Furthermore, with increasingly competitive applicants every year and inflated Step 1 scores, many programs have increased the minimum score in recent years. In 2011, the mean USMLE Step 1 score for matched orthopedic applicants was 240, and in 2016 the mean rose to 247 ($P<.001$). Similarly, the mean USMLE Step 2 Clinical Knowledge (CK) score increased from 245 in 2011 to 253 in 2016 ($P = .001$).[7]

In 2002, a survey done by Bernstein and colleagues[8] showed that in addition to USMLE Step 1 being a widely used screening criterion, orthopedic residency program directors heavily weigh class rank in medical school and participation in an away rotation at their institution. Other influencing factors mentioned in the survey include an applicant's formality during their interview, personal appearance of the applicant, and performance on ethical questions during the interview. However, when analyzing applications of US seniors who successfully matched into orthopedics, several different factors prove to be important. Applicant factors associated with increased likelihood of matching were AOA membership, USMLE Step 1 score, graduation from a top 40 National Institutes of Health–funded medical school, and the number of programs ranked.[4] Furthermore, in 2016 the average number of interviews for matched applicants was 11.5, with AOA membership having the strongest influence on interview yield.[5] This indicates a discrepancy between what program directors believe to be most important in identifying strong applicants versus what factors are predictive of matching.

Similarly, there is also a discrepancy between the most commonly used screening criteria and future resident success. Relying heavily on objective screening criteria in the form of standardized tests implies that these previous achievements are solely indicative of future success as a resident. However, there is increasing evidence that although a high USMLE Step 1 score is predictive of high performance on the Orthopedic In-Training Examination (OITE), it is not predictive of interpersonal skills, overall resident performance, or research output.[9–12] Andolsek[13] notes that USMLE Step 1 was never intended to be used as a screening tool for residencies. It was "designed as pass/fail for licensing boards to decide whether physician candidates meet minimum standards to obtain the medical licensure necessary to practice."[13] Much of the content of the examination is of little to no relevance to orthopedic surgery, but programs have not yet found a better alternative for screening in the context of a high volume of applicants.[10]

Accordingly, the National Board of Medical Examiners has opted to convert USMLE Step 1 scoring to pass/fail as early as January 2022. The utility of Step 1 as a screening tool has turned a student's performance on a single examination on a single day into a make or break milestone that limits many applicants from pursuing their preferred specialty. According to the National Resident Matching Program (NRMP) match data from 2018, 86% of US seniors applying to orthopedic surgery with a Step 1 score greater than 230 matched. Applicants with a 230 or lower matched at significantly lower rate of only 64%.[2]

When Step 1 becomes pass/fail, it is reasonable to anticipate that many programs will shift to Step 2 CK as a standardized measure for screening applicants. Although this may seem no different than using Step 1 as a screening tool, there is evidence that a higher Step 2 CK score is a better predictor of "clinical acumen" than Step 1.[4,12] Away rotations, which are already highly valued by program directors, will also likely become even more important.

The anticipated changes to Step 1 scoring are now preceded by the current global pandemic caused by SARS-CoV-2. As social distancing policies began to take place in March 2020, nearly all American medical schools temporarily canceled clerkships for third- and fourth-year medical students. The Association of American Medical Colleges Visiting Student Application Services temporarily closed in the spring of 2020, preventing students from submitting applications for away rotations. Furthermore, even for rotations that do occur, students' roles as "subinterns" or "junior interns" may be limited compared with previous years for the safety of hospital workers, patients, and the students themselves. Elective surgeries may also occur at lower rates, depending on fluctuating rates of COVID-19 cases, limiting students' exposure to a large majority of orthopedic cases.

The pandemic has also affected students' ability to take Step 2 CK and CS. Testing sites closed across the nation for months, causing thousands of students scheduled during spring and summer 2020 to miss their original examination dates forcing rescheduling of their examinations to the fall, which may occur after the initial ERAS application submission. This limits the opportunity for applicants with a lower Step 1 score to boost their performance on Step 2 CK, proving to program directors that they can perform successfully on standardized examinations.

Another effect of COVID-19 on the application process is how programs will facilitate interviews. If interviews had been scheduled for the months of March through May, programs would have had to either cancel/postpone interviews or administer them virtually. If a resurgence of COVID-19 occurs in the fall or winter of 2020 to 2021, as many public health experts are predicting, programs may have to drastically alter the interview process and interview candidates virtually.

With the most commonly used screening tool being converted to pass/fail reporting as early as 2022 and considering the unprecedented effects of the pandemic on the residency application process, residency selection committees will need to adapt and develop new ways of identifying strong applicants that fit well with their program.

PREDICTORS OF RESIDENT SUCCESS

Identifying well qualified candidates with the aptitude to become competent, caring surgeons is critical to the continued success and growth of orthopedic surgery. As Kreitz and colleagues[14] states, this "is especially true in a healthcare environment defined by quality of care, patient outcomes, and cost control."

To identify predictors of resident success, resident success must first be defined. Although this definition varies somewhat among different institutions, success metrics shared by all orthopedic residency programs are those defined by the Accreditation Council for Graduate Medical Education. According to the Accreditation Council for Graduate Medical Education, resident success incorporates mastery of six core competencies: (1) patient care, (2) knowledge for practice, (3) practice-based learning and improvement, (4) interpersonal and communication skills, (5) professionalism, and (6) systems-based practice.

One retrospective study done by Raman and colleagues[12] examined the relationship between preresidency selection factors and resident performance. Objective measures of resident performance included OITE scores and American Board of Orthopedic Surgery (ABOS) Part I scores. Subjective measures included faculty global evaluation scores and faculty rankings of residents. Overall, USMLE Step 2 CK score, the number of honors in medical school clerkships, and AOA membership demonstrated the strongest correlation with future resident performance. Step 2 scores and the number of clerkship honors positively correlated with OITE and ABOS Part I scores, whereas AOA membership correlated with higher scores on the global faculty evaluation, especially in relation to interpersonal and communication skills. On the contrary, USMLE Step 1, MCAT score, number of letters of recommendation, number of away rotations, and number of preresidency publications showed no correlation with resident success. No data were found on the relationship between quality of letters of recommendation and future success as a resident or attending.

In another retrospective study, Egol and colleagues[9] concluded that USMLE Step 1 correlates with high OITE scores and good surgical skills ratings. By comparison, higher numbers of medical school clinical honors grades correlate to higher overall resident performance, higher residency interpersonal skills grading, higher resident knowledge grading, and higher surgical skills evaluations. Similarly, Kreitz and colleagues[14] found that a high USMLE Step 1 score and Step 2 CK score positively correlate with high OITE performance. Most likely, high performance on standardized tests in medical school predicts continued high performance on standardized tests in residency.

When looking at predictive measures for research productivity, Kreitz and colleagues[14] also found that a high number of authored publications before residency indicates a high likelihood of continued research during residency. High Step 1 and Step 2 scores negatively predict research output in residency, with higher scores correlating with lower research output. However, applicants with lower Step 1 and Step 2 scores had more research experience before residency and were likely to continue research in residency. Medical school clerkship performance was also a predictor of research productivity in residency. One potential explanation for the relationship between research productivity and performance on USMLE examinations is that students with lower Step 1 and 2 scores participate in research projects to boost their applications. However, it is also possible that students who are heavily involved with research spend less time preparing for Step 1 and 2 and subsequently get lower scores. Overall, early exposure to research and greater access to research opportunities will likely increase research productivity in residency.[14]

In a retrospective analysis of neurosurgery applicants, preresidency factors that predicted future examination performance included standardized tests. Both USMLE Step 1 and Step 2 CK correlated positively with in-training examinations. However, USMLE scores were poor predictors of faculty evaluations. Aggregate rank scores, letters of recommendation, and musical talent were the strongest predictors of good faculty evaluations in residency. From these studies, one can conclude that prior examination performance predicts future examination performance, but not necessarily overall clinical competency.[11]

Grit

A concept new to the world of residency applications is "grit." In psychology, grit refers to an individual's "perseverance and passion for long-term goals."[15] Individuals that possess grit are more likely to stay motivated and determined in achieving long-term goals, despite numerous obstacles and adversities along the way. Orthopedic residency training presents various challenges, failures, and setbacks, and delayed gratification, and grit serves as an overriding factor that maintains the stamina necessary to "stay the course" amid setbacks.[16]

In a study analyzing the relationship between grit and resident well-being in a general surgery program, grit positively correlated with general psychological well-being and inversely correlated with depression and risk of attrition.[17] Attrition is a costly and disruptive problem in residency, and depression and burnout are occupational hazards with drastic effects. In the long-term, burnout leads to "erosion of professionalism, increase[ed] risk of medical errors, early retirement, and increased rate of suicidal ideation."[18] For students and residents, burnout decreases one's ability to learn continuously and impairs skills critical to educational success.[18] Because burnout often begins in medical school and residency, identifying criteria that either negatively or positively predict likelihood of burnout among applicants is critical to ensuring the development of competent residents and surgeons. According to Salles and colleagues,[17] grit is a quick and reliable measure to predict risk of depression or attrition. Because there is no evidence that individual grit significantly changes throughout years of residency, it is important to select highly gritty applicants from the beginning.

Although administering a grit assessment would have its setbacks, such as being subject to desirability bias by the applicants who fill it out, there are several objective associations that can be taken directly from applications. Camp and colleagues[19] found that increased age, decreased USMLE Step 1 score, female sex, collegiate athlete experience, and military experience correlate with a higher grit, self-control, and/or conscientiousness scores. Female applicants, AOA members, and those with higher publications are likely to have higher self-control scores. Increased self-control scores correlated with better interpersonal skills and optimal medical professionalism. Based on these positive correlations, AOA status and research productivity should continue to be used in applicant screening.

Another innovative possibility for a future screening tool is the quantitative composite scoring tool (QCST) created by the orthopedic program at Mayo Clinic. The QCST was designed in attempt to quantify many objective and subjective variables in the residency screening and selection process. It consists of 10 categories: (1) medical school reputation, (2) class rank/AOA status, (3) basic science honors grades, (4) junior year clinical clerkship honors grades, (5) Mayo orthopedic clerkship grade, (6) USMLE Step 1 percentile score, (7) undergraduate grades, (8) graduate school degrees, (9) letters of recommendation, and (10) miscellaneous/extracurricular activities. Each category has an associated point value, and the sum of all 10 category values equals the QCST score, which is used as one of four predictor variables for four outcomes assessments. Because of the inherent subjective nature of some of the QCST categories and the variability in medical school policies, such as whether a school has an AOA chapter, numeral reference tables were developed to help guide scoring. Furthermore, the medical school reputation category allows for point adjustment for applicants from schools whose grade distribution histograms show consistent grade inflation. In addition to the QCST score, the other three predictor variables analyzed were USMLE Step 1 score, AOA status, and performance in junior year core clinical clerkships. The outcomes assessments were

percentile OITE scores in final year residency, passing the ABOS written and oral examinations on first attempt, and appointment to PGY-5 chief resident associate status. Comparing the predictive value of each of the four predictor variables for the outcomes assessments, the QCST in this study had the strongest predictive value for all outcomes assessments categories. These results suggest that it is possible to develop a composite scoring tool for evaluating applicants that is an effective predictor of orthopedic resident outcomes, and that using such a tool is more effective in predicting residency outcomes compared with individual predictors, such as USMLE Step 1 scores.[20]

DIVERSITY IN ORTHOPEDICS

In 2002, the American Academy of Orthopedic Surgeons (AAOS) identified increasing women and minorities in orthopedics as a priority for the field and subsequently increased recruitment efforts.[21] More than 10 years later, a retrospective study examining the impact of the AAOS's efforts to increase diversity in orthopedics concluded that whereas diversity in medical school has increased dramatically, that is not the case in orthopedics.[22] In 2016, the AAOS census showed that orthopedic surgery continues to have the lowest proportion of female residents than any other medical or surgical specialty, including general surgery, neurosurgery, urology, and plastic surgery. Although in 2016, 47% of medical students were female, only 14% of orthopedic residents were female. When assessing orthopedic surgeons beyond residency, the discrepancy is even more profound with only 5.3% of US orthopedic surgeons being female.[21] The 2016 Association of American Medical Colleges Medical School Graduation Questionnaire showed that 82% of applicants indicated that having a role model in the field had moderate to strong influence over them choosing their specialty. Conversely, negative perceptions about the promotion of women in orthopedics have led to decreased interest in the field.[22]

Discrimination against women has also likely contributed to decreased interest in the field, as exemplified by inappropriate questions in interviews from 1970 to 2015. Thirty-eight percent of female orthopedic residency applicants who responded to the survey were asked about raising children during residency, 39% about marital or dating status, 30% about potential pregnancy in residency even for women who were single at the time, and 17% about women being inferior residents to men or referencing female physical strength.[21] A potential solution is making interview questions and format more standardized for all applicants.

Two initiatives called the Perry Initiative's Medical Student Outreach Program and the Nth Dimensions Orthopedic Summer Internship Program have shown that successful targeted outreach to first- and second-year female and underrepresented minority medical students can positively influence them to pursue orthopedics as a specialty.[22–24] The Perry Initiative's Medical Student Outreach Program is a nationwide initiative to recruit and retain women in orthopedics through outreach and mentoring. In the first 3 years of the program from 2012 to 2014, females who participated in this program were significantly more likely to apply to orthopedic surgery. Furthermore, preprogram and post-program surveys showed that the program positively influenced students' perceptions of orthopedics as a specialty.[23] The Nth Dimensions Orthopedic Summer Internship Program occurs during the summer between M1 and M2 and includes 8 weeks of orthopedic research, lectures, workshops, mentoring, and counseling. Data from 2011 to 2014 show that completion of the program significantly increased the odds of applying to orthopedic surgery residency for female medical students and underrepresented minority medical students.[24]

With most medical students today being either female or of ethnic or racial minorities, it is important for orthopedics to improve recruitment of these demographics.[25] Failure to do so will result in a significant portion of top-tier applicants gravitating toward other specialties. Furthermore, increased diversity among physicians allows physicians and trainees to learn how to interact with a diverse group of people, thus leading to better communication with and care of diverse patients.

Diversity in orthopedic residency programs "requires the commitment of the chair and program director and a focus on more than grades."[26] Achieving this goal requires effective development of pipeline programs, early exposure to the field for women and minorities, successful positive mentorship by orthopedic faculty, and focus on transforming high levels of interest in orthopedics among minority medical students into successful residency applications.[27]

SUMMARY

The landscape of the residency application process and the Match is ever-changing considering the current pandemic and future Step 1 scoring changes. The 2020 to 2021 Match will likely look different as a result of COVID-19 with limited opportunities for applicants to do away rotations and take Step 2 examinations before submitting ERAS. The transition of Step 1 scoring to pass/fail will preclude using this as a screening tool for offering residency interviews. Because so much is changing, it may also be a good opportunity to revise other aspects of the current system, such as setting a maximum number of programs to which an applicant may apply. This would ensure that students only apply to programs that genuinely interest them while also requiring programs to focus more on individual applications rather than using a screening tool to eliminate a large portion. If programs continue to use a Step 1 or Step 2 CK cutoff score for screening purposes, it would be beneficial to applicants and programs to publicize standardized score cutoffs such that applicants may decide against applying to programs whose minimum requirements they do not meet. Additional solutions could be to release interview offers on the same date and require either acceptance or rejection of the offer by a certain date, or to set a maximum number of interviews that students may attend.

Overall, although change to the current residency Match process is inevitable, the opportunities for positive change to the process are limitless. As residency applicants become more competitive, it is in the best interest of orthopedic surgery residency programs to improve current screening and selection protocols to identify predictors of future resident success. Furthermore, in an increasingly diverse world, it is critical that representation within orthopedic surgery better reflects that of the general population to provide the best possible care to patients.

CLINICS CARE POINTS

- Orthopedic surgery residency is extremely competitive. Identifying applicants who will perform well in residency and beyond is critical to the future success of the field.
- USMLE Step 1 is a commonly used screening tool for program directors to sort through residency applicants. If Step 1 becomes pass/fail, programs will have to identify new criteria for assessing applicants.
- A high USMLE Step 1 score correlates with high performance on the

Orthopedic In-Training Examination (OITE), but it is not predictive of interpersonal skills, overall resident performance, or research output.

- USMLE Step 2 Clinical Knowledge, Alpha Omega Alpha status, research experience, and clinical clerkship grades may be useful objective selection criteria for residency programs if Step 1 becomes pass/fail.
- Grit refers to an individual's resilience, "perseverance and passion for achieving long-term goals". Residency programs may benefit from identifying and selecting applicants with a high level of grit as this may lead to lower rates of burnout and depression among residents.
- Several factors associated with higher grit include AOA membership, research productivity, female sex, collegiate athlete experience, and military experience.
- The COVID-19 pandemic has limited opportunities for applicants and residency programs to interact in person via away rotations and interviews. Virtual interviews present a new challenge for programs in assessing applicants for the 2021 Match.
- Orthopedic surgery is one of the least diverse fields in medicine. Residency programs should work to increase representation of minority groups to provide the best possible care to an increasingly diverse patient population.
- Early mentorship and exposure to orthopedic surgery is necessary to increase the representation of female and minority medical students in the field.

DISCLOSURE

No conflicts of interest or funding to declare.

REFERENCES

1. Rivero S, Ippolito J, Martinez M, et al. Analysis of unmatched orthopaedic residency applicants: options after the match. J Grad Med Educ 2016;8(1):91–5.
2. National Resident Matching Program. Charting outcomes in the match: U.S. allopathic seniors. NRMP 2018. Available at: https://mk0nrmp3oyqui6wqfm.kinstacdn.com/wp-content/uploads/2019/10/Charting-Outcomes-in-the-Match-2018_Seniors-1.pdf/. Accessed April 16, 2020.
3. National Resident Matching Program. How the matching algorithm works. NRMP 2017. Available at: http://www.nrmp.org/matching-algorithm/. Accessed April 15, 2020.
4. Porter SE, Jobin CM, Lynch TS, et al. Survival guide for the orthopaedic surgery match. J Am Acad Orthop Surg 2017;25:403–10.
5. Chen AF, Secrist ES, Scannell BP, et al. Matching in orthopaedic surgery. J Am Acad Orthop Surg 2020;28:135–44.
6. Schrock JB, Kraeutler MJ, Dayton MR, et al. A cross-sectional analysis of minimum USMLE step 1 and 2 criteria used by orthopaedic surgery residency programs in screening residency applications. J Am Acad Orthop Surg 2017;25:464–8.
7. Li NY, Gruppuso PA, Kalagara S, et al. Critical assessment of the contemporary orthopaedic surgery residency application process. J Bone Joint Surg Am 2019;101(21):e114.
8. Bernstein AD, Jazrawi LM, Elbeshbeshy B, et al. An analysis of orthopaedic residency selection criteria. Bull Hosp Jt Dis 2002-2003;61(1–2):49–57.
9. Egol KA, Collins J, Zuckerman JD. Success in orthopaedic training: resident selection and predictors of quality performance. J Am Acad Orthop Surg 2011;19:72–80.
10. Porter SE, Graves M. Resident selection beyond the United States Medical Licensing Examination. J Am Acad Orthop Surg 2017;25:411–5.
11. Zuckerman SL, Kelly PD, Dewan MC, et al. Predicting resident performance from preresidency factors: a systematic review and applicability to neurosurgical training. World Neurosurg 2018;110:475–84.
12. Raman T, Alrabaa RG, Sood A, et al. Does residency selection criteria predict performance in orthopaedic surgery residency? Clin Orthop Relat Res 2016;474(4):908–14.
13. Andolsek KM. One small step for step 1. Acad Med 2019;94(3):309–13.
14. Kreitz T, Verma S, Adan A, et al. Factors predictive of orthopaedic in-training examination performance and research productivity among orthopaedic residents. J Am Acad Orthop Surg 2019;27:e286–92.
15. Duckworth AL, Peterson C, Matthews MD, et al. Grit: perseverance and passion for long-term goals. J Pers Soc Psychol 2007;92(6):1087–101.
16. Kurian EB, Desai VS, Turner NS, et al. Is grit the new fit? Assessing non-cognitive variables in orthopedic surgery trainees. J Surg Educ 2019;76(4):924–30.
17. Salles A, Lin D, Liebert C, et al. Grit as a predictor of risk of attrition in surgical residency. Am J Surg 2017;213(2):288–91.
18. Driesman AS, Strauss EJ, Konda SR, et al. Factors associated with orthopaedic resident

burnout: a pilot study. J Am Acad Orthop Surg 2020;00:1–7.

19. Camp CL, Wang D, Turner NS, et al. Objective predictors of grit, self-control, and conscientiousness in orthopaedic surgery residency applicants. J Am Acad Orthop Surg 2019;27:e227–34.

20. Turner NS, Shaughnessy WJ, Berg EJ, et al. A quantitative composite scoring tool for orthopaedic residency screening and selection. Clin Orthop Relat Res 2006;449:50–5.

21. Bohl DD, Iantorno SE, Kogan M. Inappropriate questions asked of female orthopaedic surgery applicants from 1971 to 2015: a cross-sectional study. J Am Acad Orthop Surg 2019;27:519–26.

22. Poon S, Kiridly D, Mutawakkil M, et al. Current trends in sex, race, and ethnic diversity in orthopaedic surgery residency. J Am Acad Orthop Surg 2019;27:e725–3733.

23. Lattanza LL, Meszaros-Dearolf L, O'Connor MI, et al. The Perry initiative's medical outreach program recruits women into orthopaedic residency. Clin Orthop Relat Res 2016;474(9):1962–6.

24. Mason BS, Ross W, Ortega G, et al. Can a Strategic pipeline initiative increase the number of women and underrepresented minorities in orthopaedic surgery? Clin Orthop Relat Res 2016;474(9):1979–85.

25. Association of American Medical Colleges. Total U.S. medical school enrollment by race/ethnicity (alone) and sex, 2015-2016 through 2019-2020. AAMC 2019. Available at: https://www.aamc.org/system/files/2019-11/2019_FACTS_Table_B-3.pdf. Accessed April 30, 2020.

26. Gebhardt MC. Improving diversity in orthopaedic residency programs. J Am Acad Orthop Surg 2007;15(suppl 1):S49–50.

27. Rao RD, Khatib ON, Agarwal A. Factors motivating medical students in selecting a career specialty: relevance for a robust orthopaedic pipeline. J Am Acad Orthop Surg 2017;25:527–35.

Importance of Advocacy from the Orthopedic Surgeon

Daniel E. Davis, MD, MS

KEYWORDS

- Advocacy • Political involvement • Health care policy • Legislation • Regulation

---

KEY POINTS

- The intersection of health care delivery and governmental regulations has led to the development of professional medical advocacy in the political process.
- A physician's primary purpose is to advocate on behalf of the patient, which now includes shaping the health care landscape through political advocacy.
- All orthopedic surgeons should strive to get involved with political advocacy at some level to ensure policy makers are well educated on the factors that affect the surgeons' ability to provide high-quality care.
- The American Association of Orthopedic Surgeon Political Action Committee and the Office of Governmental Regulation is a foundational resource to help guide orthopedic surgeons and get them involved in the advocacy process.

INTRODUCTION

Physicians are trained first and foremost to take care of the patient, put their interests above all else, and do so with a code of ethics that bonds the physician to the patient. It is this bond that allows physicians to earn and keep the patient's trust. There is no doubt that all of the physicians reading this enact these principles on a daily basis as the profession has done for centuries. Over the years, some physicians have taken the responsibility of this private relationship to a more public setting in which they have used their knowledge and expertise to guide and advise on broader policies that affect health care. From the beginning of the nation, individual physicians have been involved with the political process; however, it has not been until more recently that physician groups have bonded together as advocates to achieve common goals in the political process. This article highlights the history of medical advocacy and orthopedic advocacy in particular, reviews recent achievements made through orthopedic advocacy efforts, and provides tips on getting involved with advocacy efforts.

HISTORY OF MEDICAL ADVOCACY

As far back as Hippocrates there is discussion of the physician being an advocate for the patient. In the nineteenth century, Virchow emphasized the intersection of physicians and the political process. Virchow, who was a pioneer in medicine in recognizing the state of disease as an abnormal reaction of cells from their normal processes, also equated the demonstration of that disease in the individual to be a reflection of the population on a whole and the health of a society.[1] In other words, the health and state of individuals affect the health and state of the masses and vice versa. Thus, he emphasized the political forces that could alter society as the whole could help to improve the health of individuals.

This intersection of the political process and health remained mostly in the public health sector for many decades. In the United States,

---

Shoulder and Elbow Division, The Rothman Orthopaedic Institute at Thomas Jefferson University Hospital, 925 Chestnut Street, 5th Floor, Philadelphia, PA 19107, USA
E-mail address: daniel.e.davis@gmail.com

Orthop Clin N Am 52 (2021) 77–82
https://doi.org/10.1016/j.ocl.2020.08.005

it was not until The Great Society and the introduction of Medicare and Medicaid in the 1960s that the political process was truly inserted into health care delivery. Before the passage of these landmark pieces of legislation health care delivery and payments were largely focused between the doctor and the patient. It was not until post–World War II in the 1950s that employer-sponsored health insurance became more popular. This development led President Johnson to introduce government-sponsored insurance in the forms of Medicare and Medicaid to provide health coverage for the elderly and the impoverished, respectively. These plans were met with great resistance from the American Medical Association, which was one of the first examples of a large medical group getting involved in the political process through advocacy.[2]

Since the 1960s, involvement of the government in the health care delivery process has only grown. This growth led to the necessity for continued and increasing involvement of physicians and their specialty societies in the political process locally and nationally. Today, virtually every medical specialty and many subspecialties are involved in political advocacy. Topics range broadly among all physician groups but are largely focused on patients' access to care and the physician's ability to provide that care in the best way possible.

The American Academy of Orthopeadic Surgeons (AAOS) was founded in 1933 to represent those physicians who dealt with the musculoskeletal care of patients, to advocate on behalf of those patients, to provide continued education for physicians, and educate the public about prevention and treatment of musculoskeletal injuries. As it became evident that direct involvement of physicians and their interest groups in the political process was needed, the AAOS created the American Association of Orthopedic Surgeons along with the Orthopedic Political Action Committee (Orthopedic PAC) in the late 1990s. Today the AAOS and the Orthopedic PAC support and promote those issues that are important to the orthopedic community on the whole. This is done by supporting legislation and politicians who promote policies that help orthopedic surgeons take care of their patients in the best way possible.

ORTHOPEDIC ADVOCACY PROCESS

The Orthopedic PAC is led by a Committee of representatives from the AAOS Board of Specialty Societies and selected by the AAOS Committee on Committees. This larger committee is then further directed by the Orthopedic PAC Executive Committee and the Orthopedic PAC chair who help to guide policy decisions of the Orthopedic PAC. The most notable of the decisions are to develop and promote legislation that is important to orthopedic surgeons and providers of musculoskeletal care. The Orthopedic PAC Chair and Executive Committee report on an annual basis to the AAOS Board of Directors on the activities of the PAC. Finally, the AAOS Orthopedic PAC daily activities are managed out of Washington, DC, by a team of professionals with many years of experience working with politicians and their staffers through the AAOS Office of Government Relations (OGR). This team helps to coordinate efforts between the Orthopedic PAC Executive Committee and AAOS members with members of Congress.[3]

There are many ways the orthopedic surgeon can get involved in political advocacy and many good reasons to do so. Although the AAOS has a solid structure in place for political advocacy on the federal level, the interested orthopedic surgeon must also remember opportunities for advocacy on the state level. State orthopedic societies are generally well organized and connected to help the orthopedic surgeon with an interest in advocacy.

The basic levels of political involvement in any realm moving from least to most involved are: nonvoter (no involvement), voter, donor, campaigner. For those reading this article, one would assume that there is at least level of involvement through voting and a further interest involvement of political persuasion through advocacy. As orthopedic physicians with an intimate knowledge of the issues that matter to us most, building personal relationships with politicians or their staff is an effective method of advocating for change. To be able to get to the level of that type of relationship, one must climb the political pyramid, as described by Dr John Gill, Orthopedic PAC Chair, in his 2010 *AAOS Now* article.[4] As Dr Gill points out, campaign contributions are a necessary evil in the political process, especially in these times of unlimited dollars able to be raised by super PACs on the national level. However, by donating to a political campaign that donor exerts more influence than 99.9% of eligible voters in their district (in terms of US Representatives). Therefore, the easiest and most passive way of getting involved is simply to donate. This is done individually to campaigns or by donating to state PAC or the AAOS Orthopedic PAC, which then use those dollars to support a broad range of campaigns. Donations to the PAC from orthopedic surgeons have traditionally been low, but have been growing through the past decade. According to the Orthopedic PAC Annual Report in 2019, there was 18% participation of practicing orthopedic surgeons with a stated goal of increasing that number to 30% by 2020.[5] In a prospective survey study of the American Shoulder and Elbow Surgeons in 2019 by Abboud and colleagues,[6] 254 respondents reported that 110 (43%) members had donated to the Orthopedic PAC in the past year. Furthermore, 220 (87%) were willing to become more involved by being a key contact person or forming a relationship with a legislator.[6]

The next and highest level of involvement is with actively campaigning or meeting directly with local and federal representatives. This is done in a variety of ways. The simplest is a donation to a fundraiser to attend and meet the candidate and their staff. This gives you the opportunity to discuss the issues most important to you, your practice, and your community. However, although these are fantastic events to attend, they generally are focused on the candidate meeting the attendees. This can create a challenge for a worthwhile exchange of ideas; however, it provides an opportunity for an introduction. Access to these events is attained through individual donations or as a contributing member of a state orthopedic society PAC or the AAOS Orthopedic PAC. Additionally, many practices across the country and state specialty societies have creating advocacy divisions that give those practices and societies the opportunity to form relationships with representatives. The final and most intimate way to build a relationship with your local representative is to set up a meeting in your home district. On a personal note, this is something I have done to meet the US Representatives in my districts where I practice and live. This has given our group the chance to show them our practice locations, discuss our goals as orthopedic surgeons, and receive their feedback on pertinent issues. I have found this a great way to build rapport and trust with politicians to be able to have an open and honest discussion of issues at hand.

PAST ORTHOPEDIC ADVOCACY ACCOMPLISHMENTS

Before discussing current issues at the time of this writing, it is useful to discuss past accomplishments of the AAOS Orthopedic PAC and the efforts put forth by the staff of the OGR. The accomplishments listed next happened at the federal and state level and include change in legislation and regulatory mandates through 2018 and 2019.

Federal Legislation

- Passage of the Sports Medicine Licensure Clarity Act, which was a piece of legislation that originated from the AAOS and was advocated through to Congress for more than 5 years.[7] This legislation provides legal protection for sports medicine doctors caring for their athletes across state line and helps to provide readily available care to athlete patients from the physicians who know them best.
- Advocated on behalf of changes made in the 2018 Bipartisan Budget Act, which included clarifications to the Merit-based Incentive Payment System (MIPS) program and repeal of the Independent Payment Advisory Board that was created through the Affordable Care Act.
- Participated in including important verbiage in the SUPPORT Patients and Community Act focused on opioid control. The AAOS ensured provisions that will require electronic prescribing of controlled substances and provide Centers for Disease Control and Prevention grants to states to improve their Prescription Drug Monitoring Programs to help protect patients from the dangers of prescription opioid medication.

Federal Regulations

- Accomplished enacting rule changes to Centers for Medicare and Medicaid Services (CMS) guidelines for total knee arthroplasty, which had been taken off the inpatient-only list.[8] The rule change allows for surgeons to make the final decision for setting of care to that which best aligns with the patients' needs.
- Effectively helped to delay the changes proposed by CMS in evaluation and management codes and continues to be actively involved in planning a better strategy for changes moving forward.

State Advocacy Measures

- South Carolina Orthopedic Association and the AAOS Health Policy Action Fund found success with the South Carolina

Supreme Court in protecting the integration of physicians with physical therapy programs.[9]

- Massachusetts Orthopedic Association was successful in advocating the reformation of state policy to allow expansion of ambulatory surgery centers, which help provide patients with high-quality, more convenient access to care.
- Similar to the Sports Medicine Licensure Clarity Act, multiple states with the support of local orthopedic associations signed laws allowed traveling sports medicine doctors to practice medicine across state lines as long as they maintain active licensure in their home state.
- Pennsylvania Orthopedic Society advocated for the passage of legislation that limits the time period that health insurance companies could retroactively deny claims to a period of 24 months.
- Texas Orthopedic Association effectively advocated for legislation that changes the screening process for scoliosis to be in line with the latest literature. The passage of this legislation and enactment of this screening will serve as a template for national changes for the betterment of children and appropriate scoliosis screening and treatment.

ONGOING ISSUES IN ORTHOPEDIC ADVOCACY

Although the AAOS OGR and the Orthopedic PAC has been successful in advocating for achieving significant changes on a state and federal level, there are an ever growing number of political issues that are important to the practicing orthopedic surgeon. The areas of importance that the AAOS focuses on are constantly being updated on the AAOS Advocacy Web site.[10] At the time of this writing the issues currently being discussed include the following:

- Access to quality of care for patients, which includes discussions on liability reform, graduate medical education, registries, and research funding
- Physician burden relief in the form of health information technology reform and antitrust reform
- Physician ownership and ancillary services
- Payment reform including Medicare, CMS, private payors, and quality issues

Further details with more time-sensitive updates are always available through the AAOS Advocacy Web site. Additionally, for the orthopedic advocate who wants to make it to the top of the advocacy pyramid and form relationship with your local representative there are "Congressional One-Pagers," which provide succinct summaries of all these issues. These are useful handouts to provide legislators and their staff.

STARTING EARLY: ADVOCACY IN RESIDENCY

There are ample resources available to the orthopedic surgeon interested in being an advocate on behalf of patients and the profession. As political influence in health care has only grown over the decades, so too have the opportunities for health care providers grown to exert their political influence. No matter the stage in one's career, there are always options for getting involved in political advocacy in orthopedics. From residents to established orthopedic surgeons in large and small practices alike, there are ample opportunities for involvement.

Although many orthopedic residents may have an interest in the political process, few probably think they have the ability to take that interest and apply it, but they are mistaken. Although the main tenants of a successful advocate are money and time (two things orthopedic residents are short on), there are increasing opportunities built into training programs to bypass these hurdles and allow residents to get involved. The first hurdle of money is one that the leaders of the Orthopedic PAC have come up with creative solutions to promote involvement for orthopedic residents in training. First is a lower cost for residents to become members of the PAC's Capitol Club. The Capitol Club is a donor group of PAC members who have given $1000 or more per year to the Orthopedic PAC. Recognizing the burden this creates for residents, the Futures Capitol Club was created with a minimum donation of $100 per year for those in residency. This comes with all of the perks of a full Capitol Club membership. These include invitations to events at the Academy annual meeting and National Orthopedic Leadership Conference with members of Congress, opportunities to attend local fundraising events and trips, and the chance to hand deliver PAC donations to local candidates or sitting members. Another opportunity for residents and their programs to gain recognition is to have 100% resident donation participation to the PAC, even if it is just $1 per resident. This grows notoriety of the program with the PAC and the Executive Committee.[11]

The second issue of time is frequently dependent on availability within one's residency program. Although time is the one resource of which more cannot be made, many programs offer elective time or time outside of clinical responsibilities that can be used for interests in advocacy. This time is effectively used by using the resources of the Orthopedic PAC, your state orthopedic societies, or faculty mentors. Frequently any combination of these options have established avenues in which an early advocacy experience is gained. Faculty mentors are a great first step because they have connections and resources available to be able to invite the interested resident to a fundraiser or a visit with a policy maker at the state or federal level. Direct communication with one's state society is another easy outlet with each state offering different levels of participation for residents. Finally, the Orthopedic PAC has multiple opportunities in which residents can be involved. Membership in the Capitol Club comes with many excellent benefits to allow early involvement. Interested residents who are willing to commit more time and energy to early advocacy can apply for the Resident Advocacy Fellowship through the AAOS.[12] This year-long fellowship is available for PGY-3 and PGY-4 residents to apply and involves advanced time working with the OGR learning more about legislation and health policy. One week of time in Washington, DC, is required and presentations at the National Orthopedic Leadership Conference, webinars, and advocacy promotion to other residents.

ADVOCACY DURING THE COVID-19 PANDEMIC

Being an active participant in the political process involves relationship building through face-to-face interaction. In early 2020, the novel SARS-Coronavirus-2 (SARS-CoV-2) began spreading throughout the world in a pandemic-type fashion. When the epidemic reached the United States in late February and early March of 2020 Americans were faced with a significant change to their normal day to day activities. Restrictions began with new terms, such as "social distancing" and stay at home orders. This transitioned to the complete shutdown of businesses in many parts of the country including elective surgery bans to conserve hospital resources. Face-to-face interactions, large group meetings, and in-person office visits were canceled and replaced with videoconferences and the rapid expansion of telemedicine.

Political advocacy played a large role in this process and the way in which it was accomplished needed to happen in a much different way. Relationships that had been built before the pandemic played a large role in advocacy efforts moving forward. Many action items were taken care of from the government and insurance companies on the outset, such as the relaxation of rules related to telehealth visits. Many other aspects required intervention from advocacy groups, such as ensuring Medicare advance payments were made and providing payroll protection for medical practices.

Furthermore, the actual advocacy process was turned upside down, further extenuated by the fact that 2020 was a major election year. Normally, fundraisers would have been scheduled on a regular basis to meet candidates and incumbents. However, with the inability to travel and meet in person, many fundraising efforts were transitioned to teleconference format. The entire pandemic situation thus limited the ability and motivation of the individual donor to continue to donate. Additionally, although PACs were left with decreased donations, they maintained a broader ability to donate versus the individual donor. Therefore, this highlights the importance of maintaining a close connection with a state orthopedic society PAC and the AAOS Orthopedic PAC.

SUMMARY

The intersection of health care and politics has been a decades long relationship that has only grown more intense and comingled with time. Although it is not the inherent nature of most physicians to insert themselves in the political process, the argument can be made that it is a necessary aspect of one's career to be sure the voices of the physician are heard. Physicians have always been advocates for patients since the beginning of the profession. Although the root of patient advocacy is the doctor-patient relationship and providing the best care to each individual patient, the ability of the physician to do so is greatly affected by the system in which they practice. In the United States, that system is strongly connected with government entities that legislate, regulate, and many times pay for the care provided. Therefore, an intimate knowledge of the political process and relationships with policymakers involved gives the physician the know-how and ability to be sure their voices are heard to be able to provide the best possible care for their patients.

CLINICS CARE POINTS

- Orthopedic surgeons can be involved in the political process as an advocate for those issues that affect their ability to practice medicine and deliver quality care to patients.
- Advocacy involvement occurs on many levels from donating individually, to orthopedic political action committees locally and nationally, or creating and maintaining relationships with lawmakers.
- Participation in the advocacy process for orthopedic surgeons traditionally is low but has been increasing steadily.
- A larger percentage of surgeons have an interest in forming relationships with government members, which is facilitated through state societies and the AAOS Orthopedic PAC.

DISCLOSURE

The author is a contributing member to the AAOS Orthopedic PAC, the Pennsylvania Orthopedic Society PAC, and the Rothman Orthopedic Institute PAC, a member of the AAOS Orthopedic PAC Advisor's Circle.

REFERENCES

1. Mackenbach JP. Politics is nothing but medicine at a larger scale: reflections on public health's biggest idea. J Epidemiol Community Health 2009;63(3): 181–4.
2. Medicare, fair pay, and the AMA: the forgotten history | health affairs [Internet]. Available at: https://www.healthaffairs.org/do/10.1377/hblog20150910. 050461/full/. Accessed Jul 1, 2020.
3. Advocacy - American Association of Orthopaedic Surgeons [Internet]. Available at: https://www.aaos.org/advocacy/. Accessed Jul 1, 2020.
4. AAOS now July 2010: getting to the top of the political pyramid [Internet]. Available at: https://www.aaos.org/aaosnow/2010/jul/advocacy/advocacy6/. Accessed Jul 1, 2020.
5. OrthoPAC releases 2019 annual report [Internet]. Available at: https://aaos.org/aaosnow/2020/may/advocacy/advocacy04/. Accessed Jul 2, 2020.
6. Abboud JA, Jamgochian GC, Romeo AA, et al. A prospective study assessing the political advocacy of American shoulder and elbow surgeons members. J Shoulder Elbow Surg 2019;28(4):802–7.
7. Federal legislative wins - American Association of Orthopaedic Surgeons [Internet]. Available at: https://www.aaos.org/advocacy/advocacy-accomplishments/federal-legislative-wins/. Accessed Jul 1, 2020.
8. Federal regulatory wins [Internet]. Available at: https://www.aaos.org/advocacy/advocacy-accomplishments/federal-regulatory-wins/. Accessed Jul 1, 2020.
9. State advocacy accomplishments - American Association of Orthopaedic Surgeons [Internet]. Available at: https://www.aaos.org/advocacy/advocacy-accomplishments/state-advocacy-wins/. Accessed Jul 1, 2020.
10. Federal advocacy issues - American Association of Orthopaedic Surgeons [Internet]. Available at: https://www.aaos.org/advocacy/federal-advocacy-issues/. Accessed Jul 1, 2020.
11. AAOS now November 2015: resident involvement in the orthopaedic PAC [Internet]. Available at: https://www.aaos.org/aaosnow/2015/nov/advocacy/advocacy3/. Accessed Jul 1, 2020.
12. Resident advocacy fellowship - American Association of Orthopaedic Surgeons [Internet]. Available at: https://www.aaos.org/advocacy/get-involved/resident-advocacy-fellowship/. Accessed Jul 1, 2020.

Moving?

Make sure your subscription moves with you!

To notify us of your new address, find your **Clinics Account Number** (located on your mailing label above your name), and contact customer service at:

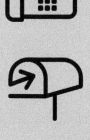

Email: journalscustomerservice-usa@elsevier.com

800-654-2452 (subscribers in the U.S. & Canada)
314-447-8871 (subscribers outside of the U.S. & Canada)

Fax number: 314-447-8029

Elsevier Health Sciences Division
Subscription Customer Service
3251 Riverport Lane
Maryland Heights, MO 63043

*To ensure uninterrupted delivery of your subscription, please notify us at least 4 weeks in advance of move.

Printed and bound by CPI Group (UK) Ltd, Croydon, CR0 4YY

08/05/2025

01864700-0011